MAN'S SUPREME INHERITANCE

Conscious Guidance and Control in
Relation to Human Evolution
in Civilization

THE WORLD FAMOUS CLASSIC
BY THE ORIGINATOR OF
THE ALEXANDER TECHNIQUE

BY

F. MATTHIAS ALEXANDER

WITH AN INTRODUCTORY WORD BY
PROFESSOR JOHN DEWEY

First Edition 1910
Second Edition 1941
Third Edition 1946
Reprinted 1946
This edition 2019

Table of Contents

PREFACE TO NEW EDITION

(London, 1945)

IT is not strange that the thoughts of all of us tend now in the direction of *change*. It would be queer indeed if this were not so, for we are all thinking the same thing and asking the same question: "How is it possible for the world to have drifted into the horrible condition in which it finds itself today?" Or, if we are more honest with ourselves, we put the question a little differently: "How could we and all the other good people in the world have allowed things to get into this dreadful mess?"

But there is another question, a more important question— one that men have asked themselves during every crisis since time began: "What must we do to be saved... where, when the horror stops, must we *begin* to make a change to prevent a recurrence?" And always the answers given to this question have left the problem unsolved, as each new dreadful crisis proves.

Yet there *is* an answer, a magnificently simple and effective answer. But man has been too blind to see, too deaf to hear. Desperately, and far afield, he continues to search for the magic key of his deliverance while he holds the very key in his own hand. It is what man *does* that brings the wrong thing about, first within himself and then in his activities in the outside world, and it is only by *preventing* this *doing* that he can ever begin to make any real change. In other words, before man can make the changes necessary in the outside world, he must learn to know the kind of doing he should prevent in himself, and the HOW of preventing it. Change must begin in his own behaviour.

But whereas many others seem to be exercised these days by what a reviewer recently called "this murky matter of human behaviour," they offer no solution to the problem of *how* this "murky matter" can be changed. Miss Dorothy Thompson made this point in the New York *Herald Tribune* recently, where she wrote:

"The only problem in the world to-day that is totally unsolved is what to do with the behaviour of the human race.... The behaviour of the human race is what this war is really about.... (It is) the only problem not even potentially solved."

Matthias Alexander

Sensitive to the rapidly growing interest in the *HOW of change in human behaviour* (the theme of this and all my other books), and remembering that no less an authority than Professor John Dewey had written in the Introduction to *Constructive Conscious Control of the Individual* that therein, as in these pages, is

> "demonstrated a new scientific principle with respect to *the control of human behaviour* as important as any principle that has ever been discovered in the domain of external nature,"

my publishers have suggested that I set down as best I can some of the Vital questions to which the reader will find an answer in this book, questions which stem from the very root of the problem of behaviour—the fact, almost always overlooked when the *how* of improving human behaviour is discussed, that *a human being functions as a whole* and can only be fundamentally changed *as a whole*. It is in the light of this fact that the technique described in this book has real significance.

Here, then, are some of the important problems relating to the control of human behaviour to which the reader can find solutions in this book:

1. Why living in a quickly changing environment has been a stumbling-block in the way of man's development and progress.
2. Why Physical-culture and present educational methods are based upon a wrong principle.
3. Why the education of the "whole child" is not possible under educational methods based upon the present principle.
4. Why Relaxation Exercises do more harm than good.
5. Why man can no longer depend on his feelings alone as a compass to guide him on the sea of life.
6. Why, in any attempt to make necessary changes in himself, man would need to do what *feels wrong* in order to *be right*.
7. Why the habit of *endgaining* is probably the most persistent and impeding habit he needs to overcome in seeking to make changes in himself or others.
8. Why the method of *direct approach* to a problem of change in behaviour so constantly fails to bring about the desired end, and why the *means whereby* to an end should depend on an

indirect procedure.
9. Why man fails so often to put his good ideas into practice, especially when he tries hardest to do so.
10. Why so many apparently *good* results of following certain methods prove in the long run to be *bad* results, and why so-called cures turn out to be merely palliatives.
11. Why it can be stated that the theory and practice set down in this book are based upon *a new principle,* and so provide a new and reliable basis for the diagnosis of human behaviour.
12. Why, last but most important of all, the use of the *inhibitory processes* is the necessary first step in the reconditioning of human behaviour.

"Systematized common sense" was the phrase once used by a reviewer in summing up his opinion of this book. The review must have been seen by many people because that phrase as applied to this book has come back to me many times in the intervening years. The original edition of *Man's Supreme Inheritance* was first published in 1910. A greatly enlarged edition was published eight years later. Thirty-five years is a ripe age for such a book, and ere this age is reached by most books they are either out of date or out of print. Not so with *Man's Supreme Inheritance.* The demand for it has continued despite war and the horrors of war. It was selling as well just before the war as when it was first published. The same holds true of all my other books. Referring to these in Part III of his book, *The Nature of Disease,* J. E. R. McDonagh, F.R.C.S., writes: "Alexander's books differ from all others in that they indicate not only the tonic (of criticism) but the actual remedial and preventive measures. The basis of the technique is the complete interdependence between the mind and the body, without which there can be no co-ordination of the whole organism named ' man.'" One critic, trying to explain the vitality of these books over so long a time, said: "They are books not for a day or a year, but for all time." Whether or not that be true is something only time can tell. But this much can certainly be said of them: they convey that knowledge of the working of the self that man needs in order to learn to control his behaviour—control or change it, that is, so that it fits in with his environment, no matter in what age, or in response to what stimulus, no matter how unfamiliar

Matthias Alexander

or how disconcerting. There is no other way for man to escape the grim hazards of his fear of the unknown.

Ever since the subject first took hold of the minds of men, the methods advocated for changing and controlling human behaviour have been legion. Good results, moreover, have been claimed for all of them. But why, if these results were anything more than palliative, are conditions in the world what they are to-day? In one of the chapters in this book, the one dealing with ' Evolutionary Standards," I warned of the danger that man's mania for gaining his ends, no matter by what means, would ultimately lead to world-wide disaster and degradation. I also explained why educational endgaining methods for quick results would stimulate war-mongering and result in those so trained becoming a menace to society and to themselves. What I have feared has come to pass. But the history of man is a long, long history, and it is never too late to change. Those who are seriously concerned with the best way of making changes in educational methods (using the word education in its widest sense) will find it well worth while to study the chapter referred to above.

The history of my discovery, or rather rediscovery, of the primary control which makes it possible for man consciously to change and improve his behaviour is told elsewhere in this book, and in the early chapters of *The Use of the Self.* But there is one phase of the technique and its history which I should like to stress at this time. It relates to the way in which the nature of behaviour is determined by the *speed* of response (reaction) to stimuli.

There came a time, early in my career, when I became aware that I was wasting my energy; wasting it, because my too1 quick reaction was a serious stumbling-block to me in practically everything I tried to do. How well I remember the words of an old man, the dearest friend of my younger days, "the more hurry, the less speed," and the kindly yet tormenting question of my mother and father, who would often ask me, "Why don't you think before you speak or act?" On one occasion I remember I retorted angrily that it was easy enough for them to ask that question, but impossible for me to answer it. The objective proof that this "impossible" was rendered possible by subsequent experience can be found in *The Use of the Self.*

When *Man's Supreme Inheritance* first appeared, its message was received with considerable doubt and prejudice, and the warning it conveyed of individual shortcomings, impending world strife, and destruction was scoffed at. The message has since been accepted, and with the advance of time the range of its acceptance widens. This gives me much satisfaction because I believe that man can escape from the serious situation in which he finds himself only by facing the bitter truth that "The fault, dear Brutus, is not in our stars but in ourselves..." I am reminded here of an old fable retold by the late Rudyard Kipling at a gathering in London. As I remember it, it went as follows:

The younger gods had offended against the holy law and were waiting for judgment in the Great Hall of Destiny. The elder god pondered long on a fitting punishment and finally gave his verdict. But the younger gods only smiled at one another and made no protest. Whereupon the elder god thundered: ' Be not so light-hearted. You shall suffer this punishment for infinite time, unless you can discover the secret that will gain your release. But I warn you, this secret is safely hid.'

At this, the younger gods cried out: ' Oh where, most merciful one, shall we begin to look? All things are known to the gods. What more must we find out? Besides, being gods, who is there with power greater than ours to help us? Surely our crime deserves not a punishment so severe? ' At this the Great Hall echoed with the laughter of the elder god. 'The secret should not be hard to find,' he answered. 'I have hidden it within you. Look there!' And he roared with laughter at his own jest."

Since this book was first published, innumerable references to the theory and practice advocated in it have been made in books, pamphlets, scientific reports, and letters of appreciation. The variety of the fields of reference indicates the wide scope of possible application. Listed below is a brief summary of some of these references:

IN EDUCATION
Professor John Dewey: Foreword to present book and Introductions to *Constructive Conscious Control* and *The Use of the Self.*

Aldous Huxley: *Ends and Means, Eyeless in Gaza.*

Matthias Alexander

P. B. Ballard, M.A.: *A.B.C. of Algebra, Things I Cannot Forget.*

IN MEDICINE
J. E. R. McDonagh, F.R.C.S.: *The Nature of Disease.*

Peter Macdonald, M.D.: Presidential Address to the Yorkshire Branch of the British Medical Association, *British Medical Journal,* December 1926.

A. Rugg-Gunn, F.R.C.S.: *F. Matthias Alexander and the Problem of Animal Behaviour.*

IN PHYSIOLOGY AND ANATOMY
G. E. Coghill, Biologist and Professor of Comparative Anatomy: Author of *Anatomy and the Problems of Behaviour* (Cambridge). See Appreciation in *The Universal Constant in Living,* by F. Matthias Alexander.

Andrew Murdoch, M.B., CM.: *The Function of the SubOccipital Muscles. The Key to Posture, Use, and Functioning.* Mungo Douglas, M.B.: *Reorientation of the Viewpoint upon the Study of Anatomy.*

IN SPORT
Sir E. Holderness: In a review of *Constructive Conscious Control of the Individual* showing the application of the technique to golf. John Duncan Duncan: *Conscious Control in Golf.*

IN CHEMISTRY
Thomas D. Hall, B.A., M.Sc.: Presidential Address, "Some Accomplishments of the Chemist," delivered to the members of the South African Chemical Institute.

IN SOCIOLOGY
Anthony M. Ludovici: *Man—An Indictment,* and *The Truth About Childbirth.*

In 1937 nineteen distinguished members of the medical profession in England urged, in the columns of the *British Medical Journal,* that my technique should be included in the curriculum for the training of medical students.

The subject-matter of this book paved the way to the

establishment of the F. Matthias Alexander Trust Fund School in Kent, England, with the Earl of Lytton, K.G., Sir Lynden Macassey, Dr. Peter Macdonald and myself as Trustees. Because of the war, the school and staff were in America, and through the kindness of the American Unitarian Association its work was carried on at the Whitney Homestead, at Stow, Mass. The school will be reopened in England as soon as conditions permit.

I am pleased to be able to name, among those who have studied the technique with me as private pupils, the following:

THE EARL OF LYTTON

PROFESSOR JOHN DEWEY

SIR STAFFORD AND LADY CRIPPS

MR. AND MRS. G. BERNARD SHAW

MR. AND MRS. ALDOUS HUXLEY

J. E. R. MCDONAGH, F.R.C.S.

PROFESSOR G. E. COGHILL

LADY RHONDDA

P. B. BALLARD, M.A.

COL. R. SMITH BARRY

A. RUGG-GUNN, F.R.C.S.

PETER MACDONALD, M.D

SIR RICHARD REES

SIR LYNDEN MACASSEY

SIR ADRIAN BOULT

MR. ROBERT DONAT

MISS MARIE NEY

DR. ANDREW MURDOCH

DR. AND MRS. MUNGO DOUGLAS

DR. JOHN SHIRLEY, M.A., HEADMASTER, KING'S SCHOOL, CANTERBURY, ENGLAND

THE LATE ARCHBISHOP OF CANTERBURY

REV. J. H. WEATHERALL, M.A., PRINCIPAL, MANCHESTER COLLEGE, OXFORD

I have often been asked the question: "Does it take long to learn the technique?" To answer this in a general way is rather difficult because so much depends on the make-up, the ideas, and the beliefs of the individual pupil. But what I wrote in 1910 still holds true:

"It is my belief, confirmed by the research and practice of nearly twenty years, that man's supreme inheritance of conscious guidance and control is within the grasp of anyone who will take the trouble to cultivate it.   That it is no esoteric doctrine or mystical cult, but a synthesis of entirely reasonable propositions that can be demonstrated in pure theory and substantiated in common practice.... "I t is essential that the peoples of civilization should comprehend the value of their inheritance, that outcome of the long process of evolution which will enable them to govern the uses of their own physical mechanisms.... This triumph is not to be won in sleep, in trance, in submission, in paralysis, or in anaesthesia, but in a clear, open-eyed, reasoning, deliberate consciousness and apprehension of the wonderful potentialities possessed by man-kind, the transcendent inheritance of a conscious mind."

F. MATTHIAS ALEXANDER.
16 Ashley Place, Westminster,
London.

PREFACE TO FIRST EDITION

(London, 1910)

AMONG my intimates I once numbered a boatman known as Old Sol, or to his familiars just Sol, without the courtesy title, for he was not notably old. I could not say whether his name was an abbreviated form of Solomon or not, nor if it were, whether the longer name was baptismal or conferred in later years as a tribute to his undoubted wisdom. I have thought it possible that the name was not an abbreviation at all, but it was certainly descriptive of my friend's habit of optimism in regard to the weather. For the Cockney oarsman who doubtfully contemplated the weather conditions on the upper Thames, Sol was unwavering in his encouragement. His certainty that the weather would clear and the sun come out was so inspiring that the pale-faced Londoner cheerfully faced the most unpromising outlook, and started out on his uncertain course upstream, buoyed with a beautiful confidence in Old Sol's infallibility. But for me and for his other intimates, regular clients whose custom was not dependent on the chances of a fine week-end, Sol had another method. In answer to the usual question, "Well, Sol, what's it going to do?" he would first look up into the sky, then step to the edge of the landingstage and study as much of the horizon as was within his limit of vision. After this careful survey he would deliver his opinion judicially, and I rarely found him at fault in his prophecy.

Facing my critics, lay and professional, I wish at the outset to disclaim the methods by which Sol invigorated the casual amateur. I am not prophesying unlimited sunshine for every one, without regard to conditions. In this book no mention will be found of royal roads, panaceas, or grand specifics. I have attempted rather to treat every reader as Sol treated his intimates. I have looked into the sky and made a careful survey of the horizon. It is true that I have seen an ideal and the promise of its fulfilment, but my deductions have been drawn with patient care from signs which I have studied with diligence; if I am an optimist, it is because I see the promise of fair weather, and not because I wish to delude the unwary. And with this I will lay down my metaphor and come to a practical statement.

I know that I shall be regarded in many quarters as a revolutionary and a heretic, for my theory and practice, though founded on a principle as old as the life of man, are not in accord with, nor even a development of, the tradition which still obtains. But in thus rejecting tradition I am, happily, sustained by something more than an unproved theory. Moreover, on this firm ground I do not stand alone. Though my theory may appear revolutionary and heretical, it is shared by men of attainment in science and medicine. On a small scale I have made many converts, and in now making appeal to a wider circle I am upheld by the knowledge that what I have to say can no longer be classed as an isolated opinion.

Not that I should have hesitated to come forward now, even if I had been without support. During the past thirteen years I have built up a practice in London which has reached the bounds of my capacity. This work has not been done by any advancement of a wavering hypothesis. I have had cases brought to me as the result of the failure of many kinds of treatment, of rest cures, relaxation cures, hypnotism, faith cures, physical-culture, and the ordinary medical prescriptions, and in the treatment of these cases, in my own observations, and in the appreciation of the patients themselves, I have had abundant opportunity to prove to my own satisfaction that in its application to present needs my theory has stood the test of practice in every circumstance and condition.

That the limits imposed by the present work render it woefully inadequate I am quite willing to admit, but the necessity for a certain urgency has been forced upon me, and I have deemed it wiser to outline my subject at once rather than wait for the time when I shall be ready to publish my larger work. Indeed, when I think of the material even now at my command, of the wonderful and ever-increasing list of illustrative cases that have passed and are still passing through my hands, it seems to me that this preliminary treatise might well grow, like Frazer's *Golden Bough,* from one volume to twelve. In the present volume, however, I must confine myself to the primary argument and to indicating the direction in which we may find physical completeness. In the work which will follow I shall deal with the detailed evidence of the application of my theory to life, of cases and cures, and all the substance of experience.

And there are many reasons why I should hesitate no longer in making my preliminary appeal, chief among them being the appalling physical deterioration that can be seen by any intelligent observer who will walk the streets of London or New York, for example, and note the form and aspect of the average individuals who make up the crowd. So much for the surface signs. What inferences can we not draw from the statistics? To take three instances only: What of the disproportionate and apparently undeniable increase in the cases of cancer, appendicitis, and insanity?[1] For that increase goes on despite the fact that we have taken the subject seriously to heart. Now I would not fall into the common fallacy of *post hoc ergo propter hoc,* and say that because the increase of these evils has gone hand-in-hand with our endeavours to raise the standard by physical-culture theories, relaxation exercises, rest cures, and *hoc genus omne,* therefore the one is the result of the other; but, lacking more definite proof on the first point, I do maintain that if physical-culture exercises, etc., had done all that was expected of them they must be considered a complete failure in the checking of the three evils I have instanced.

Are these troubles, then, still to increase? Are we to wait while the bacteriologist patiently investigates the nature of these diseases, until he triumphantly isolates some characteristic germ and announces that here, at last, is the dread bacillus of cancer? [2] Should we even

---

[1] The following Table from "Statistics and Tables," in *Health and Social Welfare* (1944-1945), edited by Lord Horder, is significant in this connection.

Table to show the increase in Cancer over the past 100 years.
Death rates per million living:

1851-60	326
1861-70	396
1871-80	484
1881-90	610
1891-1900	767
1901-10	867
1911-20	928
1921-30	985
1931-40	974

[2] Investigators, however, almost unanimously incline now to the theory that the cause of cancer is a morbid proliferation of the cells not due to the primary influence or isolation of alien bacteria.

then be any nearer a cure? Could we rely on inoculation, and even if we could, what is to be the end? Are we to be inoculated against every known disease till our bodies become depressed and enervated sterilities, incapable of action on their own account? I pray not, for such a physical condition would imply a mental condition even more pitiable. The science of bacteriology has its uses, but they are the uses of research rather than of application. Bacteriology reveals a few of the agents active in disease, but it says nothing about the conditions which permit these agents to become active. Therefore I look to that wonderful instrument, the human body, for the true solution of our difficulty, an instrument so inimitably adaptable, so full of marvellous potentialities of resistance and recuperation, that it is able, when properly used, to overcome all the forces of disease which may be arrayed against it.

In this thing I do not address myself to any one class or section of the community. I have tried in what follows to avoid, so far as may be, any terminology, any medical or scientific phrases and technicalities, and to speak to the entire intelligent public. I wish the scheme I have here adumbrated to be taken up universally, and not to be restricted to the advantage of any one body, medical or otherwise. I wish to do away with such teachers as I am myself. My place in the present economy is due to a misunderstanding of the causes of our present physical disability, and when this disability is finally eliminated the specialized practitioner will have no place, no uses. This may be a dream of the future, but in its beginnings it is now capable of realization. Every man, woman, and child holds the possibility of physical perfection; it rests with each of us to attain it by personal understanding and effort.

F. MATTHIAS ALEXANDER.
16 Ashley Place, Westminster, London.

INTRODUCTORY WORD

MANY persons have pointed out the strain which has come upon human nature in the change from a state of animal savagery to present civilization. No one, it seems to me, has grasped the meaning, dangers, and possibilities of this change more lucidly and completely than Mr. Alexander. His account of the crises which have ensued upon this evolution is a contribution to a better understanding of every phase of contemporary life. His interpretation centres primarily about the crisis in the physical and moral health of the individual produced by the conflict between the functions of the brain and the nervous system on one side and the functions of digestion, circulation, respiration, and the muscular system on the other; but there is no aspect of the maladjustments of modern life which does not receive illumination.

Frank acknowledgment of this internecine warfare in the very heart of our civilization is not agreeable. For this reason it is rarely faced in its entirety. We prefer to deal with its incidents and episodes as if they were isolated accidents and could be overcome one by one in isolation. Those who have seen the conflict have almost always proposed as a remedy either a return to nature, a relapse to the simple life, or else flight to some mystic obscurity. Mr. Alexander exposes the fundamental error in the empirical and palliative methods. When the organs through which any structure, be it physiological, mental, or social, are out of balance, when they are unco-ordinated, specific and limited attempts at a cure only exercise the already disordered mechanism. In "improving" one organic structure, they produce a compensatory maladjustment, usually more subtle and more difficult to deal with, somewhere else. The ingeniously inclined will have little difficulty in paralleling Mr. Alexander's criticism of "physical-culture methods" within any field of our economic and political life.

In his criticism of return or relapse to the simpler conditions from which civilized man has departed Mr. Alexander's philo sophy appears in its essential features. All such attempts represent an attempt at solution through abdication of intelligence. They all argue, in effect, that since the varied evils have come through development of conscious intelligence, the remedy is to let intelligence sleep, while the pre-intelligent forces, out of which it developed, do their work.

Matthias Alexander

The pitfalls into which references to the unconscious and subconscious usually fall have no existence in Mr. Alexander's treatment. He gives these terms a definite and real meaning. They express reliance upon the primitive mind of sense, of unreflection, as against reliance upon *reflective* mind. Mr. Alexander sees the remedy not in a futile abdication of intelligence in order that lower forces may work, but in carrying the power of intelligence farther, in making its function one of positive and constructive control. As a layman, I am incompetent to pass judgment upon the particular technique through which he would bring about a control of intelligence over the bodily organism so as not merely to cure but to prevent the present multitudinous maladies of adjustment. But he does not stop with a pious recommendation of such conscious control; he possesses and offers a definite method for its realization, and even a layman can testify, as I am glad to do, to the efficacy of its working in concrete cases.

It did not remain for the author of these pages to eulogize self-mastery or self-control. But these eulogies have too frequently remained in the hortatory and moralistic state. Mr. Alexander has developed a definite procedure, based upon a scientific knowledge of the organism. Popular fear of anything sounding like materialism has put a heavy burden upon humanity. Men are afraid, without even being aware of their fear, to recognize the most wonderful of all the structures of the vast universe—the human body. They have been led to think that a serious notice and regard would somehow involve disloyalty to man's higher life. The discussions of Mr. Alexander breathe reverence for this wonderful instrument of our life, life mental and moral as well as that life which somewhat meaninglessly we call bodily. When such a religious attitude towards the body becomes more general, we shall have an atmosphere favourable to securing the conscious control which is urged.

In the larger sense of education, this whole book is concerned with education. But the writer of these lines was naturally especially attracted to the passages in which Mr. Alexander touches on the problems of education in the narrower sense. The meaning of his principles comes out nowhere better than in his criticisms of repressive schools on one hand and schools of "free expression" on the other. He is aware of the perversions and distortions that spring from that unnatural suppression of childhood which too frequently passes for school training. But he is equally aware that the remedy is not to be sought through a blind reaction in abolition of all control except such as the movement's whim or the accident of environment may provide. One gathers that in this country Mr. Alexander has made the acquaintance of an extremely rare type of "self-expressive" school, but all interested in educational reform may well remember that freedom of physical action and free expression of emotion are means, not ends, and that as means they are justified only in so far as they are used as conditions for developing power of intelligence. The substitution of control by intelligence for control by external authority** not the negative principle of no control or the spasmodic principle of control by emotional gusts, is the only basis upon which reformed education can build. To come into possession of intelligence is the sole human title to freedom. The spontaneity of childhood is a delightful and precious thing, but in its original naive form it is bound to disappear. Emotions become sophisticated unless they become enlightened, and the manifestation of sophisticated emotion is in no sense genuine self-expression. True spontaneity is henceforth not a birthright, but the last term, the consummated conquest, of an art—the art of conscious control to the mastery of which Mr. Alexander's book so convincingly invites us.

JOHN DEWEY.

PART I
MAN'S SUPREME INHERITANCE

CHAPTER 1 - FROM PRIMITIVE CONDITIONS TO PRESENT NEEDS

"Our contemporaries of this and the rising generation appear to be hardly aware that we are witnessing the last act of a long drama, a tragedy and comedy in one, which is being silently played, with no fanfare of trumpets or roll of drums, before our eyes on the stage of history. Whatever becomes of the savages, the curtain must soon descend on savagery forever."—J. G. FRAZER.

THE long process of evolution still moves quietly to its unknown accomplishment. Struggle and starvation, the hard fight for existence, working with fine impartiality, remorselessly eliminate the weak and defective. New variations are developed and old types no further adaptable become extinct, and thus life fighting for life improves towards a sublimation we cannot foresee. But at some period of the world's history an offshoot of a dominant type began to develop new powers that were destined to change the face of the world.

Speculation as to what first influenced that strange and wonderful development does not come within the province of this treatise, but I should like in passing to point out that the theory and practice of my system are influenced by no particular religion nor school of philosophy, but in one sense may be said to embrace them all. For whatever name we give to the Great Origin of the Universe, in the words of a friend of mine "we can all of us agree... that we mean the same thing, namely, that high power within the soul of man which enables him to will or to act or to speak, not loosely or wildly, but in subjection to an all-wise and invisible Authority." The name that we give to that Authority will in no way affect the principles which I am about to state. In subscribing to them the mechanist may still retain his belief in a theory of chemical reactions no less than the Christian his faith in a Great Redeemer. But through whatever influence these new powers in man came into being I maintain that they held strange potentialities, and, among others, that which now immediately concerns us, the potentiality to counteract the force of

1

Matthias Alexander

evolution itself.

This is, indeed, at once the greatest triumph of our intellectual growth and also the self-constituted danger which threatens us from within. Man has arisen above nature, he has bent circumstance to his will, and striven against the mighty force of evolution. He has pried into the great workshop and interfered with the machinery, endeavouring to become master of its action and to control the workings of its component parts. But the machine has yet proved too intricate for his complete comprehension. He has learned gradually the uses of a few parts which he is able to operate, but they are only a small fraction of the whole.

What, then, is man's position to-day, and what is his danger? His position is this. In emerging from the contest with nature he has ceased to be a natural animal. He has evolved curious powers of discrimination, of choice, and of construction. He has changed his environment, his food, and his whole manner of living. He has inquired into the laws which govern heredity and into the causes of disease. But his knowledge is still limited and his emergence incomplete. The power of the force we know as evolution still holds him in chains, though he has loosened his bonds and may at last free himself entirely. Thus we come to man's danger.

Evolution—a term we use here and elsewhere in this connection as that which is best understood to indicate the whole operation of natural selection and all that it connotes—has two clearly denned functions; by one of these it develops, by the other it destroys. By an infinitely slow action it has developed such wonders as the human eye or hand; by a process somewhat less tedious it allows any organ that has become useless to perish, such as the pineal eye or (in process) the vermiform appendix, and, if we can estimate the future course, the teeth and hair.

By the change he has effected in his mode of life, man is no longer necessarily dependent on his physical organism for the means of his subsistence, and in cases where he is still so dependent, such as those of the agriculturist, the artisan, and others who earn a living by manual labour, he employs his muscles in new ways, in mechanical repetitions of the same act, or in modes of labour which are far removed from those called forth by primitive conditions. In some ways the physical type which represents the rural labouring population is,

2

in my opinion, even more degenerate than the type we find in cities, and mentally there can be no comparison between the two. The truth is that man, whether living in town or country, has changed his habitat and with it his habits, and in so doing has involved himself in a new danger, for though evolution may be cruel in its methods, it is the cruelty of a discipline without which our bodies become relaxed, our muscles atrophied, and our functions put out of gear.

The antagonism of conscious as opposed to natural selection [3] has now been in existence for many thousands of years, but it is only within the last century or less that the effect upon man's constitution has become so marked that the danger of deterioration or decay has been thrust upon the attention, not only of scientific observers, but of the average, intelligent individual. No examination of history is necessary in this place to set out a reason for this comparatively sudden realization of physical unfitness. Briefly, the civilization of the past hundred years has been unlike the many that have preceded it, in that it has not been confined to any single nation or empire. In the past history of the world an intellectual civilization such as that of Egypt, of Persia, of Greece, or of Rome, perished from internal causes, of which the chief was a certain moral and physical deterioration which rendered the nation unequal to a struggle with younger, more vigorous, and—this is important— wilder, more natural peoples. Thus we have good cause for believing that the danger we have indicated, though as yet incipient only, was a determining cause in the downfall of past civilizations. But we must not overlook the fact that destructive wars and devastating plagues held sway in the earlier history of mankind, and whilst the latter acted as an instrument

It should, however, be clearly understood in this connection that certain laws of natural selection must, so far as we can see, always hold good; and it would not be advisable to alter them even if it were possible. For example, that curious law may be cited which ordains the attraction of opposites in mating and so maintains nature's average. The attraction which a certain type of woman has for a certain type of man, and vice versa, is, in my opinion, a fundamental law, and any attempt to regulate it would be harmful to the race. This, however, is

[3] For a further statement of one aspect of heredity, see Chapter VI of this book.

no argument against the regulation of prevention of marriages between the physically and mentally unfit. of evolution in destroying the unfit, the former, by decreasing the population, threw a burden of initiative and energy on the remnant, necessitating the use of active physical qualities in the business of all kinds of production.

Now the conditions have altered. Greater scientific attainments in every direction than have ever been known have combated, and will probably in the future overcome, the devastating diseases which have decimated the populations of cities, whilst a higher ethical ideal constantly tends to oppose the horrible and repugnant barbarism of war which, with the spread of civilization even to the peoples of the Orient, becomes to our senses more and more fratricidal, a fight of brother against brother.

A hundred years ago Malthus, a prophet if not a seer, recognized our danger, and within the past quarter of a century a dozen theorists have proposed remedies less stringent than those advocated by Malthus, but almost equally futile. Among the theorists are those perhaps unconscious reactionaries who advocate the simple life, by a return to natural food and conditions, in endlessly varying ways. To them in their search for natural foods and conditions we would point out that countless generations separate us from primitive man, a lapse of time during which our functions have become gradually adapted to new habits and environment, and that if it were possible by universal agreement for the peoples of Europe to return instantly to primitive methods of living, the effect would be no less disastrous than the reversal of the process, the sudden thrusting of our civilization upon savage tribes whereby, to quote one or two recent examples only, the aborigines of North America, New Zealand, and Japan (the Ainu tribes) have become, or are rapidly becoming, extinct.

When therefore we point out man's power of adaptability in this connection, the emphasis is thrown on the slowness with which that adaptability is passed on to our descendants and on the relative permanence of the new powers acquired. For our purpose the argument remains good whether we admit or deny the inheritability of acquired characteristics, our point being that in either case the process is necessarily a slow one, though it is plainly more rapid if the hypothesis be true.[4]

From the savage to the civilized state, man passed, as I say, so slowly that the passing in the early stages caused neither difficulties nor changes sufficiently marked to force themselves on our recognition. In other words, the subject of these changes was unconscious of them, and the habit of depending on these sensory appreciations ("feeling tones," or "sense of feeling "), dominant by right in the savage or subconsciously directed state, remained firmly established in the civilized experiences, so that to-day man walks, talks, sits, stands, performs in fact the innumerable mechanical acts of daily life, without giving a thought to the psychical and physical processes involved.

It is not surprising that the results have proved unsatisfactory. The evils of a personal bad habit do not reveal themselves in a day or in a week, perhaps not in a year, a remark that is also true of the benefits of a good habit. The effects of the racial habits I am now describing have gone on unnoticed for untold centuries. But in the last hundred years the evil has become so marked that its effect has at last forced itself upon our attention. The failure of subconscious guidance in modern civilization is now being widely admitted, and the consideration of this fact has led a few to the logical conclusion that conscious guidance and control is the one method of adapting ourselves not only to present conditions, but to any possible conditions that may arise. We have passed beyond the animal stage in evolution and can never return to it.

For these reasons it becomes necessary, if we would be consistent, to reject at once all propositions for improving our future well-being which can by any possibility be described as reactionary. Even in this brief *resume* of man's history one tendency stands out clearly enough, the tendency to advance. When that first offshoot from a dominant type began to develop new powers of intellect, a form was initiated which must either progress or perish. Atavism must be counteracted by the powers of the mind, and reaction is a form of atavism. No return to earlier conditions can increase our knowledge of the secret springs of life, or aid our formulation of world-laws by

---

[4] For fuller explanation, see Chapter VII

the understanding of which we may hope to control the future course of development.

The physical, mental, and spiritual potentialities of the human being are greater than we have ever realized, greater, perhaps, than the human mind in its present evolutionary stage is capable of realizing. And the present world crisis surely furnishes us with sufficient evidence that the familiar processes we call civilization and education are not, alone, such as will enable us to come into that supreme inheritance which is the complete control of our own potentialities. One of the most startling fallacies of human thought has been the attempt to inaugurate rapid and far-reaching reforms in the religious, moral, social, political, educational, and industrial spheres of human activity, whilst the individuals by whose aid these reforms can be made practical and effective have remained dependent on subconscious guidance with all that it connotes. Such attempts have always been made by men or women who were almost completely ignorant of the one fundamental principle which would so have raised the standard of evolution, that the people upon whom they sought to impose these reforms might have passed from one stage of development to another without risk of losing their mental, spiritual, or physical balance.

For in the mind of man lies the secret of his ability to resist, to conquer, and finally to govern the circumstance of his life, and only by the discovery of that secret will he ever be able to realize completely the perfect condition of mens sana in corpore sano.

CHAPTER II - PRIMITIVE REMEDIES AND THEIR DEFECTS

"... Having heard that Henry Taylor was ill, Carlyle rushed off from London to Sheen with a bottle of medicine, which had done Mrs. Carlyle good, without in the least knowing what was ailing Henry Taylor, or for what the medicine was useful."—*Life of* TENNYSON.

THE danger of that mental, nervous, and muscular debility, which is the outcome of the conditions resulting from the trend of our development, has been widely recognized during the past fifty years, and we must turn aside for a moment to consider certain phases of its treatment as indicated by the well-known and widely applied terms "physical-culture," "relaxation," and "deep-breathing."

With regard to "physical-culture," it must be clearly understood that I do not allude to any one system or practice, but speak in the widest terms; terms which are applicable alike to the most primitive forms of dumb-bell exercise, or to the most elaborate series of evolutions designed to counteract the effect of a particular malady. But lest my application of the term be misunderstood, I will explain that where I write "physical-culture" thus, between inverted commas and with a hyphen, I mean it to stand for "a series of *mechanical* exercises, simple or complicated, designed to strengthen a bodily function by the development of a set of muscles or of the complete system of muscles "; but where I use the words physical-culture, currently and without a hyphen, I denote a general system for the improvement of the entire physical economy by a just co-ordination and control of all the parts of the system, particularly excluding any method which tends to the hypertrophy of any one energy without regard to the balance of the whole.

In the first place it will be recognized, from what I have already said, that the whole theory upon which the present "physical-culture" school is based is but another aspect of that reversion to nature which we have stigmatized as a form of atavism. It is an attempt to stiffen the new garment of our intellectual development by lining it with the old fabric of so-called "natural exercise." "Physical-culture," as defined, is what one might term the obvious, uninspired method which naturally presents itself as a remedy for the ills arising from an artificial condition. The logic of it is of the simplest, and proceeds from the major premise that bodily defects arise from the disuse and misuse of muscles and energies in an artificial civilization, which muscles and energies in a natural state would be continually called upon to provide the means of livelihood.

From this it seems obvious to argue that if we contrive an artificial mechanical means of exercising these muscles for, let us say, one, two, or three hours a day, they will resume their natural functions, and so— The lacuna cannot be satisfactorily filled. If we carry on the argument to its logical conclusion the fallacy is made evident. For the method arising from this argument creates civil war within the body. There is no co-ordination, and the outcome must be strife. This point will be at once made clear by an instance which must be taken to represent a broadly typical case, an allegory rather than a special example of particular application.

Let us take for example the case of John Doe, whose work keeps him indoors from 9 a.m. to 6 p.m., and makes a very urgent call upon his mental and nervous powers. By the time he is thirty-five, possibly five or ten years earlier, John Doe is suffering from anaemia, indigestion, nervous debility, lassitude, insomnia, heart weakness, and heaven only knows what other troubles. His bodily functions are irregular, his muscular system partly atrophied and unresponsive, his nerves irritated, and his general condition—there is really no better word— "jumpy."

Incidentally I must add that his mind is inoperative in many directions. He has a bad mental attitude towards the physical acts of everyday life. For him his body is a mechanism, the intricate workings of which he never pauses to examine, but which he drives or forces through a certain series of evolutions similar in kind to those it has always performed within his experience. When this mechanism fails, it has to be forced on again by tonics and stimulants or given a "rest," which is followed by a return to the old methods of propulsion.

However, John Doe, who has already postponed far too long his search for a remedy, at last takes a course of "physical-culture," although his time is severely limited, and his exercises are confined to an hour or two morning and evening. At first he may say that he feels a wonderful benefit and probably advises every friend he meets in the City to follow his example. I am quite willing to grant that Doe may be benefited, I will even admit that if he continues his exercises it is possible he may not fall back into the same state of nervous prostration into which he fell originally, but the point I wish to make quite clear is that his cure did not in itself possess the elements of permanence. It was merely a tinkering or botching-up of the fabric of his body. For if we consider his case from a purely detached standpoint, we must see that Doe attempted to develop two systems or modes of life which could not in the nature of things work harmoniously together. On the one hand, for two, three, or four hours a day he was occupied in mechanically developing his muscular system without any reference to the *manner* in which he drove his machine, stimulating and accelerating the supply of blood, which therefore required increased oxygenation or reinforced lung power; in brief, he was exercising those functions and energies which in a primitive state would have been called upon during the greater part of his waking life to supply him with food. On the other hand, for the remaining twelve hours or so, during which he was engaged in his profession, in the eating of meals or in reading, in playing indoor games or in similar sedentary occupations, the newly developed powers were being neglected and a call was being made upon the old nervous energies and centres of control. John Doe's physical body thus had two existences, excluding the natural condition of sleep, one fiercely active, muscular, dynamic, the other sedentary, nervous, static.

These two existences are not correlated, they are antagonistic; they do not mutually support each other, they conflict. John Doe's body becomes the scene of a civil war, and the heart, lungs, and other semi-automatic organs are in a state of perpetual readjustment to opposing conditions, as they are called upon to support one side or the other in the perpetual combat. Such a condition cannot tend in the long run to the improvement of mankind as a whole.

For, as I shall show later,[5] in the case of John Doe and in all parallel cases, the consciousness of the person concerned is not changed in regard to the use of the muscular mechanism. Even if he exercise for six hours daily, on taking up his ordinary occupations once more he will immediately revert to the same muscular habits he has already

---

[5] For a fuller analysis of this, see "Habits of Thought and Body" of this volume.

acquired in connection with such occupations. For it is clear that John Doe has a wrong mental attitude towards the uses of his muscular mechanism in the acts of everyday life. He has been using muscles to do work for which they were never intended, whilst others, which should have been continuously employed, have remained undeveloped, inert, and imperfectly controlled. We may say in truth that he is suffering from mental and physical delusions with regard to the uses of his body. To mention but one of many instances of his lack of recognition of the true uses and functions of his muscular system, we shall notice that whenever he thrusts his head forward or throws it back his shoulders always accompany the movement in either direction, this movement of the shoulders being entirely unconscious and made without any recognition of the fact that they are being moved. Now in this condition of mental and physical delusion, the unfortunate man tries to do something with these mechanisms which he is unable to control, hoping that by the mere performance of certain physical exercises he can restore his body to a condition of perfect physical health.

It may be well at this point, seeing that I have admitted the possibility of some preliminary benefit to John Doe from his first experience of the "physical-culture" exercises, to show more in detail why that benefit was not maintained. The fact is that when this man realized the seriousness of his digestive troubles he was simply recognizing a symptom and not a primary cause or causes of his increasing disorders. A proper psychophysical examination would have revealed bad habits in his waking and sleeping moments which tended more or less to reduce his intra-thoracic capacity to a minimum; such a minimum is not only harmfully inadequate, but also renders due functioning of the vital organs practically impossible.

Incidentally it may be of value to consider what this condition of minimum intra-thoracic capacity really means and to note some of the influences upon the whole organism. For as this thoracic cavity contains many of the vital organs, all are the abdominal viscera directly or indirectly influenced by its capacity. Minimum thoracic capacity means that the organs within the thorax are harmfully compressed and that the heart and lungs do not get a proper chance to function adequately. A harmful strain is thrown upon the heart, the lungs are not adequately employed or sufficiently aerated, and the lung tissue deteriorates. The proper distribution of the blood is interfered with because of the undue accumulation in the splanchnic area, to the detriment of the lung supply. As the lungs are the chief distributors of blood, it will be understood that this condition of minimum thoracic capacity interferes with the circulation and general nutrition. The respiratory processes are employed in sucking in air instead of creating a partial vacuum in the lungs by a co-ordinated thoracic expansion which will give atmospheric pressure its opportunity.[6] There is an undue intra-abdominal pressure and harmful flaccidity of the abdominal muscles, which means dropping of the viscera, imperfect functioning of the liver, kidneys, bladder, etc., stagnation in the bowels and irritation and distention of the colon, intestines, etc.; in other words, indigestion, constipation, and all the concomitant disorders and general impairment of the vital functioning. Let us, for a moment, think of the thoracic and abdominal cavities as one fairly stiff oblong rubber bag filled with different parts of a working machine which are interrelated and interdependent, and which are held in position by their attachment to the different parts of the inner surface of this bag. We will then suppose, for the sake of our illustration, that the circumference of the inner upper half of this bag is three inches more than that of the lower half. As long as this general capacity of the bag is maintained the working standard of efficiency of the machinery is indicated as the maximum. Let us then, in our mind's eye, decrease the capacity of the upper part of the bag and increase that of the lower half until the inner circumference of the latter is three inches more than the former. We can at once picture the effect on the whole of the vital organs therein contained, their general disorganization, the harmful irritation caused by undue compression, the interference with the natural movement of the blood, of the lymph, and of the fluids contained in the organs of digestion and elimination. In fact we find a condition of stagnation, fermentation, etc., causing the manufacture of poisons which more or less clog the mental and physical organism, and which constitutes a process of slow poisoning.

Now to revert to the experience of John Doe. I have already stated that when he first tried physical exercises at home or in the

---

[6] For a fuller explanation, See Chapter VII.

gymnasium as a remedy for his digestive disorders, he experienced
a sense of relief. This was only natural, seeing that he was leading a
more or less sedentary life. Why, then, was the effect of these
exercises gradually diminished until he considered the physical
treatment a comparative failure? This brings us to the point of real
interest. The fact is that any increased amount of exercise does give
a sense of relief to those who lead sedentary lives, but unfortunately
this sense of relief is too often a delusive mental exaggeration of the
real changes in the right direction. It is not often a reliable register of
benefits derived which make for permanent relief. Students of these
questions know that the man whose conditions we are analysing has
already developed debauched *kinaesthetic* systems which permit
defective registrations of different sensations or feeling-tones, and
hence it is very difficult for the person so constituted to arrive at a
reliable estimate of the extent of his improvement through such faulty
senses. We know, too, that, so far as he is concerned, the
improvement is not permanent, a fact which he readily admits.
There are scientific reasons for accepting the accuracy of this
conclusion, and I will endeavour to explain the position. Let us
admit, for the sake of our explanation, that benefits actually accrued
in various directions in the early stages of his physical exercises.
Whatever these benefits may have been, and however great they
were, I contend that it was always certain that sooner or later, if he
persisted in the physical exercises, he would gradually develop
defects which would counterbalance and finally outweigh the benefits
we have admitted.

The following are some of the reasons which support these
contentions. I shall deal more fully with them in later chapters.

1. A Defective Kinaesthetic System. Experience has proved to us
that the conditions present when he took up the exercises go hand in
hand with an incorrect and defective kinaesthetic system.

The mere performance of physical exercises could not give him
a new and correct kinaesthetic sense in connection with the use of the
mental and physical organism in his acts of everyday life.

2. Erroneous Preconceived Ideas. It is impossible for me to set
down the myriad dangers with which he is beset in consequence of
erroneous preconceptions during his daily practice on "physical-
culture" lines. The pages of a fairly large book will be necessary to do

12

even meagre justice to this subject. But I can assure my readers that this is demonstrably true and I am daily convincing the most sceptical by practical procedures.

3. Defective Sense-Registration and Delusions. This serious defect is in practice linked up with erroneous preconceptions resulting in mental and physical delusions which are farreaching and dangerous.

An Example. Take a person who, prior to re-education, has the habit of putting the head back whenever an attempt is made to put the shoulders back. Ask this person to put the head forward and keep the shoulders still, and it will be found that as a rule he fails to carry out the order, and moves his shoulders also. Ask him to put the head forward whilst the teacher holds the shoulders still, and the pupil will put the head back instead of forward.

4. Defective Mental and Physical Control. The most common form of this defective control encountered in teaching work is when the teacher wishes to move the head, or hand, or arm, or leg for the pupil, in order to give the new and correct sensation in the proper use of the parts. Experience proves that the great majority are utterly wanting in the controls necessary to enable the person to gain this experience quickly.

The teacher asks the pupil to lift his arm. He does so, but exercises an undue amount of tension. In order to give the pupil the new kins esthetic register of the correct amount of tension necessary, the teacher asks to be permitted to lift the arm for him, but as a rule the pupil acts exactly as he did when he was requested to perform the act himself.

5. Defective Inhibition. The practical teacher finds all pupils more or less hampered by lack of inhibitory control, the possession of which would make re-education and co-ordination from the pupil's standpoint comparatively easy. Consideration will show that our ordinary mode of life and the generally accepted teaching methods do not make for the development of the inhibitory powers. On the contrary, our powers in this direction rather tend to diminish, and the outward and visible signs of the serious results are everywhere for him who runs to read.

6. Self-Hypnotism. This very serious and all too common evil has not been attacked on a practical basis. People have spoken of it and written about it in a general theoretical way, much as they have done about relaxation, but with no better results on the practical side, when applied to everyday life. The self-hypnotism I am referring to is a specific self-hypnotism indulged in at a given and particular time, and is cultivated unknowingly by teachers and pupils during lessons, and frequently by both in everyday life.

People will tell you they can think better by closing their eyes. This is a prevalent form of self-hypnotism, self-deception, and produces a state of dreaming which is particularly serious because it is a harmful condition assumed consciously. The ordinary dreamer falls into this condition unconsciously.

7. *Cultivated Apprehension.* This is probably the most serious condition which we cultivate, and which has been dealt with at length in the chapter on Apprehension and Education.

8. *Prejudiced Arguments and Attempted Self-Defence.* The real weakness and shallowness of human nature is shown in this connection in a way which is uncomplimentary to our intellectual pride. The saddest fact is, that it is always intensified in the person who would be counted above the average in intellectuality by a consensus of opinion. We are all well aware that to win an argument such an one will strain his statement of his facts in the direction he desires them. His reason is so dominated by his emotions and his sense appreciation (feelingtones) that an appeal to the former is at first in vain. The majority of mankind has over-compensated in these directions, and it is for this reason that in the education and development of the child of to-day and the future, we must see to it that we relinquish all educational methods which tend to cultivate guidance and control through the emotions and the sensory appreciations (feeling-tones).

Some perception of the evils that we have thus briefly summarized has been awakened in the minds of the more earnest thinkers during the last few years, and, as a result, the systems of exercises display a clearly marked tendency towards modification. They have lessened their muscle-tensing violence, and have become, and are becoming, ever less and less strenuous physical acts. Thus we find "physical-culture" advocates who a few years ago insisted upon the use of dumbbells, and in some cases dumb-bells increasing in weight over a graduated series of exercises, now emphasizing the necessity for *gentle* exercises without even mentioning the dumb-bell, which is perhaps as good a proof as any of the truth of my contentions.

My next instance—namely, "relaxation"—is even less efficient. The usual procedure is to instruct the pupil, who is either sitting or lying on the floor, to relax, or to do what he or she understands by relaxing. The result is invariably collapse. For relaxation really means a due tension of the parts of the muscular system intended by nature to be constantly more or less tensed, together with a relaxation of those parts intended by nature to be more or less relaxed, a condition which is readily secured in practice by adopting what I have called in my other writings the position of mechanical advantage.[7] But apart from an incorrect understanding of the proper condition natural to the various muscles, the theory of relaxation, like that of the rest cure, makes a wrong assumption, and if either system is persisted in, there must inevitably follow a general lowering of vitality which will be felt the moment regular duties are taken up again, and which will soon bring about the return of the old troubles in an exaggerated form.

The last remedy mentioned at the opening of this chapter was "deep-breathing." This is a later form of "physical-culture" development, and is, in effect, a modification in the right direction.

It is the logical outcome of the perception that strenuous, forcing, muscular exercises were resulting in new and possibly greater evils than those they professed to cure. "Deep-breathing" is indeed a step in the right direction, but only a step, because, while it does not always do serious harm, and in some instances, perhaps, a certain amount of good, it does not go to the root of the matter, the eradication of defects, nor does it take cognizance of the most important factor in the. scheme of physical co-ordination.   What that radical factor is I shall explain in detail in my next chapter, but I will first briefly review the chief points of the argument as far as it has been unfolded.

In imagination we have seen man through the darkness which covers his first appearance on the earth, the early Miocene man. As we have pictured him he was a creature of simple needs and of a vigorous bodily habit, an animal in all save that spark of self-consciousness which burned feebly in his primitive, but increasing and differentiating brain. Again we have a somewhat clearer vision of him with wider powers of courage and cunning, adapting weapons to his use, and so specializing the functions of his mind through a

---

[7] See Part II, Synopsis of Claim.

long two million years, through paleolithic and neolithic periods into the age of bronze, where he has become a reasoning, designing creature, with powers of imagination and idealization, powers still turned, however, to physical uses.

And at last we reach the differentiation of man from man and class from class which marks the historical period of civilization, the period of dwelling in cities, of adaptability to new and specialized habits, of labour that makes little or no call upon the physical capacities, of food procured without energy, the period when the slow process of evolution, which has resulted in the product of a new and marvellous instrument of selfconscious, directive powers, was becoming gradually superseded by that which it had brought forth.

CHAPTER III - SUBCONSCIOUSNESS AND INHIBITION

"You can have neither a greater nor a less dominion than that over yourself."—LEONARDO DA VINCI.

WITHIN the last thirty years we have evolved a new science, the science of psychology. A generation ago psychology was subject-matter only for the philosopher, the metaphysician, the poet, or the ecclesiastic; now it is being investigated in the laboratory by tests of sensibility, reaction-times, and other responses to stimulation too technical to be explained here, tests carried out by means of elaborate and intricate instruments and machinery designed to weigh the *hidden springs of life* in the balance. The phrase I have italicized is purposely vague, for I have no wish to fall foul of a terminology or to make any *a priori* assumption which might involve me in controversial matters completely outside my province. At the same time I see clearly that some convenient phrase will become necessary, and I will therefore adopt one which is at least familiar, and within certain limits descriptive enough—namely, the "subconscious self."

It may seem strange that one should look to any such formally organized science as modern psychology, to a science that is working in a laboratory with mechanical appliances, for any elucidation of a question which has for so long been regarded as strictly within the domain of the priest. But science, as Tyndall said, is only another name for common sense, and a little consideration will show that the postulate I have insisted upon—namely, the growth and progress of intellectual control —demands that this admirable quality of common sense or reason should be applied to the elucidation of this all-important problem.

Unhappily, psychology, from which we hope so much, is as yet in its infancy, and the few attempts that have been made, such as those of the late Professor Münsterberg, to apply the theories of the laboratory and the classroom to the practical work of the world, cannot be said to have produced any results worth considering. In any case I must transcend the present limits of academic psychology in this consideration of the subconscious.

The concepts which have grown up round this term, the "subconscious self," are in many cases curiously concrete in form. Much error has sprung from that earnest and well intentioned work of the late F. W. H. Myers, *Human Personality and its Survival after Bodily Death.* Mr. Myers pictured an entity within an entity, and his work, though inductive in form, was *a priori* in method, for he had formed the conception of a subjective personality taking shape within an objective, material shell, and had controlled his evidence to a definite, preconceived end.

The fallacies of Myers have been exposed again and again. His argument is intrinsically unsound, and when put to the test of newer knowledge his hypothesis fails to explain the fact. But because Myers' conception was so graphic and credible it took a strong hold upon the popular imagination, a hold which in the eight years following the publication of *Human Personality* has not become weakened in the minds of a great number of people, full though these years have been of discovery and new knowledge. It is for this reason that I have reverted to Myers' conception of the subconscious, or as he called it, the "subliminal self," inasmuch as I wish it to be clearly understood from the outset that I use the term "subconscious self" to denote an entirely different concept. Indeed, any one who has followed my argument to this point must have inferred the trend of my purpose—namely, that as the intellectual powers of man extend, we progress in the direction of *conscious control.* The gradual control of evolution by the child of its production has pointed always to this end, and by this means, and by this alone, can the human race continue in the full enjoyment of its physical powers without forfeiting a fraction of its progressive intellectual ideal.

It will inevitably be asked at this stage what I mean when I speak of the "subconscious self," and I must therefore answer that question to the best of my ability, even though I have to leave for a moment the limits of proved fact to tread on the wider ground of hypothesis. I do not propose, however, to overburden my theory with the detail of evidence, and what follows must therefore be taken as an inclusive statement, much of which I could prove conclusively in a larger work, whilst the unproved remnant must necessarily await confirmation from the researches of future investigators in the domains of psychology. In the first place, then, we must see not only that the subconscious self is not a possession peculiar to man, but that it is in fact more active, in many ways more finely developed, in the animal world. Among some animals the consciousness of danger is so keen that we have attributed it to prescience. The fear of fire in the prairies, of flood, or of the advance of some natural danger threatening the existence of the animal, is evidenced far ahead of any signs perceptible by human senses, and as we cannot, except sentimentally, attribute powers of conscious reasoning to the animal world, it is evident that this "foreknowledge" is due to a delicate co-ordination of animal senses. Again, we see that animals which have not had their powers dulled by many generations of domestication make the majority of their movements, as we say, "instinctively." They can judge the length of a leap with astonishing accuracy, or take the one certain chance of escape among the many apparent possibilities open to them without an instant's hesitation, and as these powers are evidenced in some cases within a few hours or minutes after the birth of the animal, they are admittedly not the outcome of experience.

The whole argument for the evidence of the possession of a subconscious self by animals can be elaborated to any length, and depends on facts of observation made over a long period of time. The few examples I have here cited merely illustrate that side of the question which throws into prominence the point of what we may call abnormal powers, or powers which seem to transcend those of human reason so far as it has been developed. It is this appearance of transcendent qualities in the human subconsciousness which misled Myers, who did not pause to apply his allegory of the subconscious entity to the animal world. Such an application would have tended to prove that the "soul" (for that is what Myers really intended, however carefully he may have avoided the actual word) of the animal was more highly developed than that of man.

In the second place, however, we are confronted with the unquestionable fact that the subconsciousness can be "educated" below the plane of reason. Acts very frequently performed become so mechanical that they can be repeated without any sense of conscious awareness by the operator. The pianist, after constant rehearsals, will perform the most intricate passage while his attention is engaged with an entirely unrelated subject—although it is particularly worthy of remark in this connection, that when such an art as the performance of music falls temporarily into such an automatic repetition, the connoisseur will instantly recognize the loss of some quality—generally spoken of as "feeling"—in the rendering. Again, it appears that in some cases a more or less permanent impression may be made upon the subconsciousness by casual suggestions, often related to fear, even though such suggestions be, in some cases, the result of a single experience. A nervous hysterical subject, already far too willing to submit to the guidance of emotion and what he or she fondly believes to be "instinct" or "intuition," may be so harmfully impressed in this way as to develop any of the many forms of "phobia," which are, as the suffix correctly implies, forms of morbid terror. These are but two instances of the "education" of the subconsciousness below the reasoning plane, but a dozen others will suggest themselves to the reader out of his own experience. The important point is the fact that the phase of being with which we are dealing becomes, as we progress through life, a composite of animal instincts and habits acquired below the plane of reason either by repetition or by suggestion. But before I leave this general conception of the subconsciousness, I must emphasize the fact that up to this point we share the qualities of the subconscious mind with the animal kingdom. For in the lower organisms no less than in that of humanity, this subconsciousness can be educated. The observations of naturalists now confirm the belief that the young of certain birds—the swallow has been particularly instanced—are *taught* to fly by the parent birds; whilst any one who has trained a dog will know how such a trick as "begging" for food may become so habitual as to appear instinctive.

So much for general definition; I come now to the point which marks the differentiation of man from the animal world, and which is first clearly evidenced in the use of the reasoning, intellectual powers of inhibition.

Now it is evident that in the earlier stages of man's development the inhibition of the subconscious animal powers was frequently a source of danger and of death. Reason, not as yet sufficiently instructed and far-seeing, was an inefficient pilot, and sometimes laid the ship aback when she would have kept before the wind if left to herself. To abandon the metaphor, the control was imperfect, it wavered between two alternatives, and by rejecting the guidance of instinct it suffered, it may be, destruction. But the necessity for conscious control grew as.' the conditions of life came to differ ever more and more from those of the wild state. This, plainly, was due to many causes, but chiefly to the limitations enforced by the social habit which grew out of the need for co-operation.

This point must be briefly elaborated, for it marks the birth of inhibition in its application to everyday life, and in so doing it demonstrates the growth of the principle of conscious control which, after countless thousands of years, we are but now beginning to appreciate and understand.

It is true that we have evidence of conscious inhibition in a pure state of nature. The wild cat stalking its quarry inhibits the desire to spring prematurely, and controls to a deliberate end its eagerness for the instant gratification of a natural appetite. But in this, and in the many other similar instances, such instinctive acts of inhibition have been developed through long ages of necessity. The domestic kitten of a few weeks old, which has never been dependent on its own efforts for a single meal, will exhibit the same instinct.' In animals the inherited power is there; in man also the power is there as a matter of physical inheritance, but with what added possibilities due to the accumulated experience gained from the conscious use of this wonderful force.

The first experience must have come to man very early in his development. As soon as any act was proscribed and punishment meted out for its performance, or as soon as a reward was consciously sought—though its attainment necessitated realized, personal danger—there must have been a deliberate, conscious inhibition of natural desires, which in its turn enforced a similar restraint of muscular, physical functioning. As the needs of society widened, this necessity for the daily, hourly inhibition of natural desires increased to a bewildering, extent on the prohibitive side. There grew up first "taboos," then the rough formulation of moral and social law, and on the other hand a desire for larger powers which encouraged qualities of emulation and ambition.

Among the infinite diversity of these influences, natural appetites and the modes of gratifying them were ever more and more held in subjection, and the subconscious self or instinct which initiated every action in the lower animal world fell under the subjection of the conscious, dominating intellect or will. And in this process we must not overlook one fact of supreme importance—viz., man still progressed physically and mentally. It is therefore clear that this control acquired by the conscious mind broke no great law of nature, known or unknown, for, if this acquired control had been in conflict with any of those great, and to us as yet incomprehensible forces which have ruled the evolution of species, the animal we call man would have become extinct, as did those early saurian types which failed to fulfil the purpose of development and perished before man's first appearance on this earth.

Before we attempt, then, any exact definition of the subconscious self we must have a clearer comprehension of the terms "will," "mind," and "matter," which may or may not be different aspects of one and the same force. More than two thousand years of philosophy have left the metaphysicians still vaguely speculating as to the relations of these three essentials, and personally, I am not very hopeful of any solution from this source. The investigation, though still in its infancy in this form, has taken the shape of an exact science, and it is to that science of psychology as now understood that I look to the elucidation of many difficult problems in the future. Without touching on the uncertain ground of speculative philosophy, I will try, however, to be as definite as may be with regard to my conception of the subconscious self.

In the first place, great prominence has been given to the conception of the subconscious self as an entity within an entity, by the claim made for it that it has absolute control of the bodily functions. This claim depends for its support on the evidence of hypnotism and of the various forms of autosuggestion and faith-healing. Under the first heading, we have been told that under the direction of the hypnotist the ordinary functions of the body may be controlled or superseded, as for instance that a wound may be formed and bleed without mechanically breaking the skin,[8] or that a wound

---

[8] Cf. *Hypnotism,* by Albert Moll. Good cases of suppuration, blistering, and bleeding, as the result of suggestion without any preliminary abrasion of the skin, are those supplied by the records of Professor Forel's experiments at the Zurich Lunatic Asylum. These experiments were conducted on the person of a nurse who is described

may be healed more rapidly than is consistent with the ordinary course of nature. Under the second heading, which includes all forms of self-suggestion, we have had examples of what is known as stigmatization,[9] or the appearance on the bodies of hysterical and obsessed subjects of some imitation of the five sacred wounds. Indeed, the instances of cures which seem to our uninstructed minds miraculous, and due by inference to the power of faith, are so numerous that no special example need be cited. These and many kindred phenomena have been explained on the hypothesis that the hidden entity, when commanded by the will, is able to exert an all-powerful influence either beneficent or malignant, the obscure means by which the command may be enforced being variously described. We see at once that the conception of a hidden entity is the primitive explanation which first occurs to the puzzled mind. We find the same tendency in the many curious superstitions of the savage who turns every bird, beast, stone, and tree into a Totem, and endows them with powers of evil or of good, and discovers a "hidden entity" all of a piece with this conception of the subconscious self, in a piece of wood that he has cut from a tree, or a lump of clay that he has modelled into the rude shape of man, bird, or beast.

My own conception is rather of the unity than the diversity of life. And since any attempt to define the term Life would be presumptuous, the definition being beyond the scope of man's present ability, I will merely say that life in this connection must be read in the widest application conceivable. And it appears to me that all we know of the evolution or development of life goes to show that it has progressed, and will continue to progress, in the direction of self-consciousness.[10] If we grant the unity of life and the tendency of its evolution, it follows that all the manifestations of what we have called the "subconscious self" are functions of the vital essence or life-force, and that these functions are passing from automatic or

---

as the daughter of healthy country people, and not a hysterical subject.

[9] There is much evidence on this point, some of it conflicting, but the main fact must be considered above question.

[10] Cf. Herbert Spencer, *Education,* Chapter XI, "Humanity has progressed solely by self-instruction."

unconscious to reasoning or conscious control. This conception does not necessarily imply any distinction between the thing controlled and the control itself. This may be inferred from the use of the word "self-conscious," but the further elucidation of this side of the theory is not germane to the present argument.

Now I am quite prepared to accept as facts phenomena of the kind I have instanced, such as unusual cures effected by hypnotism, and by the somewhat allied methods of the various forms of faith-healing, but I do deny, and most emphatically deny, that either procedure is in any way necessary to produce the same or even more unusual phenomena.[11] In other words, I maintain that man may in time obtain complete conscious control of every function of the body without, as is implied by the word "conscious," going into any trance induced by hypnotic means, and without any paraphernalia of making reiterated assertions or statements of belief.

Apart from my practical experience of the harm that so often results from hypnotic and suggestive treatment, an experience sufficient to demonstrate the dangers of applying these methods to a large majority of cases, I found my objection to these practices on a broad and, I believe, incontrovertible basis. This is that the obtaining of trance is a prostitution and degradation of the objective mind, that it ignores and debases the chief curative agent, the apprehension of the patient's conscious mind, and that it is in direct contradiction to the governing principle of evolution, the great law of self-preservation by which the instinct of animals has been trained, as it were, to meet and overcome the imminent dangers of everyday existence. In man this desire for life is an influence in therapeutics so strong that I can hardly exaggerate its potentiality, and it is, moreover, an influence that can be readily awakened and developed. The will to live has in one experience of mine lifted a woman almost from the grave, a woman who had been operated upon and practically abandoned as dead by her surgeons. A passing thought flashing across a brain that had all but abandoned the struggle for existence, a sudden consciousness that her children might not be well cared for if she died, was sufficient to reawaken the desire for life, and to revivify

---

[11] Moreover, I deny that hypnotism can possibly succeed except in comparatively rare instances. It is not universal in its applicability.

a body which no medical skill could have saved.[12] But there is no need to quote instances. The fact is recognized, yet how small is the attempt made to use and control so potent a force! The same argument may be also applied to the prostration of the mind as a factor in the popular rest cures which really seek to put the mind, the great regenerating force, out of action.

Returning to my definition of the subconscious self, it will be seen that I regard it as a manifestation of the partly-conscious vital essence, functioning at times very vividly but on the whole incompletely, and from this it follows that our endeavours should be directed to perfecting the self-consciousness of this vital essence. The perfect attainment of this object in every individual would imply a mental and physical ability and a complete immunity from disease that is still a dream of the future. But once the road is pointed, we must forsake the many by-paths, however fascinating, by-paths which lead at last to an *impasse* and necessitate a return in our own footsteps. Instead of this, we must devote our energies along the indicated road, a road that presents, it is true, many difficulties, and is not straight and easy to traverse, but a road that nevertheless leads to an ideal of mental and physical completeness almost beyond our imaginings.

---

[12] 1 Two years later this woman came to me in a state of collapse, the results of the after-effects of a bad attack of pleurisy. She proved an admirable patient, and is now in perfect health. She was a magnificent instance of a case in which the power was there, finely developed, but not the knowledge which would enable her to make full use of that power.

CHAPTER IV - CONSCIOUS CONTROL

"Man one harmonious soul of many a soul
Whose nature is its own divine control." —SHELLEY.

ONE of the most recent phases of popular, as opposed to scientific, thought has been that which has endeavoured to teach the control of the mind. This teaching has been spoken of in general as the "New Thought" movement, though certain of its precepts may be found in Marcus Aurelius. This movement has had, and is still having, a considerable vogue in America, and the influence of it has been felt in England, many of the writings of its exponents having been published here within the last fifteen or twenty years. The object of the teaching is to promote the habit of "right thinking" which is to be obtained by the control of the mind. The "New Thought" teaches that certain ideas, such as fear, worry, and anger, are to be rigidly excluded from the mind and the attention fixed upon their opposites, such as courage, complacency, calm. With certain of the tendencies expressed in this movement I am in sympathy, but following the usual course of such movements, the "New Thought" is losing sight of its principle, which was, indeed, never fully grasped, and is becoming involved in a species of dogma, the rigidity of which is in my opinion directly opposed to its primary object. One of its earlier and most capable exponents, however, Ralph Waldo Trine, marked the principle with a phrase, and by naming one of his works *In Tune with the Infinite,* gave permanence to the central idea, though more recent writers in embroidering the theme have lost sight of the original thesis. Moreover, I have not found in the "New Thought" a proper consideration of cause and effect in treating the mental and physical in combination. These writings exhibit, and have always exhibited, the fallacy of considering the mental and physical as in some sense antitheses which are opposed to each other and make war, whereas in my opinion the two must be considered entirely interdependent, and even more closely knit than is implied by such a phrase.

Again, in all these writings we are confronted with one word which is dominant, and by its iteration must produce an effect on the mind of all readers. That word is "faith," and because it is so prominent and so little understood, I feel that it is essential I should give some explanation of it in the light of my own principles.

In the first place, it is perhaps hardly necessary for me to point out that faith in this connection need not be allied with any conception of creed or religion. It is true that this is the form in which we are most familiar with it in mental healing, and the associations which are grouped round the word itself very commonly induce us to connect it with the conceptions that have had such a wide and general influence on the thoughts of mankind in all stages of civilization. But we have abundant evidence now before us that in healing it is the patient's attitude of mind that is of the first importance, and that faith is every whit as effective when directed towards the person of the healer, a drug, or the medicinal qualities supposed to be possessed by a glass of pure water, as when it is directed to a belief in some supernal agency. This fact is indisputable, and it is only because the latter form of faith is so much more widespread, inasmuch as it lies at the very foundation of all religions, that this agency has effected a number of cures out of all proportion to those brought about by faith in some purely material object. What I here intend by faith, therefore, is its exercise in the widest sense and without any restriction of creed.

So far as we can analyse the effect of what we call an act of faith on the mental processes, it would seem that it is operative in two directions. The first is purely emotional. The patient, having conceived a whole-hearted belief that he is going to be delivered from his pain or disease by the means of some agency supernal or material, experiences a sensation of profound relief and joy. He understands and believes that without effort on his part he is to be cured by an apparent miracle, and the effect on him is to produce a strong, if evanescent, emotional happiness. In this we have an exact parallelism between the patient whose cure is physical and material, and the convert whose cure is spiritual. Now it is widely acknowledged by scientists and the medical profession generally that this condition of happiness is an ideal condition for the sufferer, that it is not only the most helpful condition of mind, but that it actually produces chemical changes in the physical constitution, changes which are the most salutary in producing a vital condition of the blood, and hence of the organism.

The second way in which this act of faith operates is in the breaking down of a whole set of mental habits, and in the substitution for them of a new set. The new habits may or may not be beneficial from the outset apart from the effect produced by the emotional state, which is hardly ever maintained for a long period, but even so the breaking down of the old habits of thought does produce such an effect as will in some cases influence the whole arrangement of the cells forming the tissues, and dissipate a morbid condition such as cancer.

Thus we see that this so-called act of faith is in reality purely material in its action, and there is no reason why we should have recourse to it to produce the same and greater effects. It may perhaps be asked by some objectors why we should seek to dismiss the act of faith, since it undoubtedly produces these ideal conditions in some cases. The answer is obvious. Faith-healing is dangerous in its practice and uncertain in its results. It is dangerous, because in the majority of cases its professors seek in the first place to alleviate pain. They may do this, leaving the disease itself untouched, but as I shall point out later on, in such cases the disease will continue and eventually kill the patient, even though he may be able successfully to fight the pain. Faith-healing is also uncertain in its results, because, in addition to the danger I have mentioned, it merely substitutes one uncontrolled habit of thought for another. At first the new habit, because it is new, may bring about a change to a better condition, but if it remains, it will in its turn become stereotyped, and may very well lead at last to just as morbid a condition as was induced by the old mental habit it superseded. For these reasons, which are, I think, trenchant enough, I desire most earnestly to see all the present conceptions that surround this profession of faith-healing thrown aside in order that we may arrive at a sane and reasoned process of mental therapeutics. I have touched briefly on the movement here because it emphasizes the fact that we are dimly grasping at a truth but paralysing our attempts to hold it by the premature assumption that we have it safe at last. At the same time I believe that underlying the teachings of these recent movements, "New Thought" and "Faith-healing" in general (and in these two closely allied influences I include all the offshoots and subdivisions), there is some apprehension of an essential, an apprehension which is liable to lose its grip by reason of the dogma and ritual that have grown up and tend to obscure the one fundamental.

All these sects, parties, societies, creeds—call them what you will—have a common inspiration; we need no further proof than this, that no one of the many developments from the common source is in itself complete and perfect. There is good evidence that each new development as soon as it becomes specialized is separated from its true source, becomes overelaborated, and so works its own downfall, the principle becoming absorbed and dominated by the bias of some individual mind. This is my analysis of the phenomena. It follows that what we seek is the noumenon, the reality, the true idea that underlies all these various manifestations.

Before I attempt, however, to trace out this common principle, I wish to make three statements:

I do not profess to offer a finally perfected theory, for by so doing I should lay myself open to the same arguments I have advanced against other theories of the same nature. I say frankly that we are only at the beginnings of understanding, and my own wish is to keep my theory as simple as possible, to avoid any dogma.

I do not propose, for many reasons, to consider in this place my own methods in any other connection but that of their application to physical defects, to the eradication of diseases, distortions, and lack of control, and, progressively, to the science of race-culture and the improvement of the physique of the generations to come.

I wish it to be clearly understood that this treatise is not finally definitive. I hope in the future to have many opportunities of elaborating my general thesis and of stating my experience of particular applications of my methods to peculiar cases, but I should not be true to my own principles if I were not willing to accept amendments, even perhaps to alter one or other of my premises, should new facts tend to show that I have made a false assumption in any particular. Now that I have thus cleared the ground, I will examine what I believe to be the first and greatest stumbling-block to conscious self-control—namely, "rigidity of mind." This rigidity results in a fixed habit of thought and its concomitant evils, among which is the subjection of functional and muscular habits to subconscious control.

In defining rigidity of mind, I must hark back for a moment to that suggestive phrase of Mr. Trine's, *In Tune with the Infinite,* although in the present application the rigidity I am concerned with is considered in a physical connection and does not involve interference with any non-spatial conceptions. It is rather the first half of the phrase that is here of importance, for to be "In Tune" conveys to my mind, and I wish it to convey the same meaning to others, the idea of sensitiveness to impressions and responsiveness to the touch, when "all the functions of life are becoming an intelligent harmony." In a word, I want by this phrase to suggest the idea of being openminded. For even in reading this, if the individual deliberately puts himself in opposition to my point of view, he can by no possibility hope to benefit. Wherefore I desire above all things that he or she will read at least with an open mind, form no conclusion until I have finished, and will perhaps, more particularly, subdue the interference of that great and ruling predisposition which has in the past so long impeded the advance of science, and with which I will deal in my next chapter.

Let us consider for a moment the application of rigidity of mind to physical functions. A person comes to me with some crippling defect due to the improper use of some organ or set of muscles. When I have diagnosed the defect and shown the patient *how* to use the organ or muscles in the proper way, I am always met at once with the reply, "But I can't." Let me ask any one who is reading this and who suffers in any way, whether his or her attitude to the defect they suffer from is not precisely the same? This reply indicates directly that the control of the part affected is entirely subconscious; if it were not, we should merely have to substitute the hopeful "I can" for that despondent "I can't," to remove the trouble. By *(a)* hypnotic treatment, by *(b)* faith-healing, or by (c) the application of the principles of the "New Thought," the patient in such a case would have the subconscious control influenced, either *(a)* by the mechanical means of trance and suggestion by the hypnotist, which leaves the conscious mind in exactly the original condition and merely changes, and it may be only temporarily, the habit of the subconscious control, or *(b)* and (c) by reiterated commands of the objective mind. Even if these commands have been reinforced by the influencing suggestion of the healer, they either substitute by repetition one habit for another without any apprehension by the intelligence of the true method of the exchange, or, what is quite as frequent and far more harmful, they shut out the sensitiveness to pain from the cerebral centres, and so leave the radical evil, no longer labelled by nature's warning, to work the patient's destruction in secret. Briefly, all three methods seek to reach the subjective mind by deadening the objective or conscious mind, and the centre and backbone of my theory and practice, upon which I feel that I cannot insist too strongly, is that THE CONSCIOUS MIND MUST BE QUICKENED.

It will be seen from this statement that my theory is in some ways a revolutionary one, since all earlier methods have in some form or another sought to put the flexible working of the true consciousness out of action in order to reach the subconsciousness. The result of these methods is, logically and inevitably, an endeavour to alter a bad subjective habit whilst the objective habit of thought is left unchanged. The teachings of the "New Thought" and of many sects of faith-healers set out clearly enough that the patient must think rightly before he can be cured, but they then set out, automatically, to carry out their teaching by prescribing "affirmatives" or some sort of "auto-suggestion," both of which are in effect no more than a kind of self-hypnotism, and, as such, are debasing to the primary functions of the intelligence.

I will take a simple instance from my own experience to illustrate a case in point. A patient, whom I will call X, came to me with an obstinate stammer arising from a congenital defect in the co-ordination of the face, tongue, and throat muscles. Whenever X attempted to speak he drew down his upper lip. This was the outward sign of a series of vicious acts connected with a train of muscular movements, a sign that the ideo-motor centres were working to convey a wrong guiding influence to the specific parts concerned in the act of speech. These guiding influences rendered X quite incapable of speech, and would, indeed, have had the same effect on any other individual who produced the same working of the parts concerned. To insist in such a case that X should repeat, "I can speak" or "I won't stutter," would be merely to endeavour to reach a supposed omniscient subconscious self which would counteract the evil by the exercise of some assumed and separate intelligence possessed by it. I undertook the case by appealing to X's intelligence.

Now, strange as it may seem (and I intend to treat this curious perversion in my next chapter), X's objective intelligence is not so easily reached and influenced as might appear. He has formed a muscular habit of drawing down his lip independently of his conscious control, and the line of suggestion set up by the wish to speak induces at once a reflex action of a complicated set of muscles. X has learned to do this automatically, and at first seems incapable of controlling those lip muscles when the wish to speak is initiated.

In this case my first endeavour must be directed to keeping in abeyance, by the power of inhibition, all the mental associations connected with the ideas of speaking, and to eradicating all erroneous, preconceived ideas concerning the things X imagines he can or cannot do, or what is or is not possible. My next effort must be to give X a correct and conscious guidance and control of all the parts concerned, including, of course, the lip and face muscles, and in order to obtain this control, he must have a complete and accurate apprehension of all the movements concerned. And this apprehension must precede and be preparatory to any conception of "speaking," during the application of all the guiding orders involved. In originating some new idea which is to take the place of the old idea of drawing down the upper lip, it may be necessary at first to break the old association by means of some new order, such as deliberately to draw the lip up, to open the mouth, or to make some similar muscular act previously unfamiliar in its application to the act of speaking. This new order is then substituted for the command to speak. X is told not to speak but to draw up his lip, open his mouth, etc. It will be understood that I have omitted much detail touching the interdependence of the parts concerned, but I wish here to convey the essentials of method rather than the physiological explanation of their working. It must always be remembered that Nature works as a whole and not in parts, and once the true cause of the evil is discovered and eradicated all the affected mechanisms can soon be restored to their full capacity. I may note here that X was completely cured of his stammer, and that his was a particularly obstinate case, a fact chiefly due to the confirmation of a wrong habit in early childhood.

This is an example, chosen for its simplicity, to illustrate the prime essentials of my theory, but it is capable of a very wide application, so wide that it may be applied to the working not only of the ordinary controlled muscles, but of the semi-automatic muscles which actuate the vital organs. Not many years ago an Indian Yogi was examined by Professor Max Müller at Cambridge, and we have it on the authority of the latter that this Yogi was able to stop the beating of his own heart at will and suffer no harmful consequences.

Let it be clearly understood, however, that I have no sympathy with these abnormal manifestations, which I regard as a dangerous trickery practised on the body, a trickery in no way admirable or to be sought after. The performances of the Yogis certainly do not command my admiration, and the wellknown system of breathing practised and taught by them is, in my opinion, not only wrong and essentially crude, but I consider that it tends also to exaggerate those very defects from which we suffer in this twentieth century. I have merely quoted this case of the Yogi in support of my assertion that there is no function of the body that cannot be brought under the control of the conscious will.

That this is indeed a fact and not a theory, I do claim without hesitation, and I claim further that by the application of this principle of conscious control there may in time be evolved a complete mastery over the body, which will result in the elimination of all physical defects. Certain aspects of this control and the reasons why it has not been acquired I will treat under the next heading.

CHAPTER V - APPLIED CONSCIOUS CONTROL

A CONCEPTION OF THE PRINCIPLES INVOLVED

THE term "conscious control" is one which is employed by different people to convey different conceptions. The usual conception is one which indicates specific control, such as the moving of a muscle consciously, and is practised by athletes who give performances of physical feats in public. Again, there is the conscious movement of a finger, toe, ear, or some other specific muscle or limb.

The phrase "conscious control" when used in this work is intended to indicate the value and use of conscious guidance and control, primarily as a *universal,* and secondly as a *specific,* the latter always being dependent on the former in practical procedure.

Furthermore, it is not used merely to indicate a guidance and control which we may apply in the activities of life with but doubtful precision in one or two directions only, but one which may be applied universally, and with precision in all directions, and in all spheres where the mental and physical manifestations of mankind are concerned.

Since the publication of my book, *Conscious Control,* I have received and continue to receive letters from interested readers concerning the practical application of conscious control, and also regarding my conception of the principles involved.

"It is all very well to talk of conscious control, but how are we to acquire it?" wrote one inquirer. "How far-reaching is its application?" wrote another, whilst a third remarked, "If your experience has proved that such far-reaching beneficial effects result from conscious guidance and control, your concept must be much more comprehensive than that usually accepted." "I have a friend who is cursed with a bad temper," wrote another inquirer, "and he realizes the fact. He has applied to his medical and spiritual advisers for help. They have given him a certain amount of valuable advice, but the result is far from satisfactory."

We all know of cases of men and women who eat or drink more than is good for them, and we also know that only a small minority are able to master their unhealthy desires in these directions. Examination of the misguided majority would reveal the fact that they were badly co-ordinated, and that psycho-physical conditions were present which would lead an expert to expect an overbalanced state in one direction or another, a domination of conscious reasoned control by subconscious unreasoned desire.

Such cases may be readily and successfully dealt with on a basis of conscious guidance and control in the spheres of reeducation, readjustment, and co-ordination.

To gain control where there is a tendency to over-indulgence in alcohol or food, is a very difficult problem for the ordinary human being while he remains in his badly co-ordinated condition. This is shown by the failure which succeeds failure until the unfortunate person arrives at the conclusion that it is impossible to break the habit.

He or she then drifts into the advanced stages of a condition which becomes as akin to disease as neuritis, neurasthenia, indigestion, or rheumatism. As a matter of fact these malconditions may be the immediate outcome of the indulgences before referred to.

The unfortunate fact which we must face is that such people are practically without control where these failings are concerned, and the general opinion is that these people lack willpower. In my opinion this is not really true.

Say that a man is a thief and is caught and punished. He tells his friends and relatives that he intends to reform. But does he really intend to do so? In the first instance does not the answer to this question depend on the point of view of the person concerned? Let us take as an example two brothers. The one is a thief, but the other is not, inasmuch as he has never stolen anything in his life. He would scorn such an act, but he has no hesitation in taking advantage of a friend with whom he makes an agreement. He may even fail to *realize* that he is acting unjustly towards his friend. The fact is, he is well acquainted with the details and possibilities of the business concern which this agreement represents. He is aware of his superior knowledge and he deliberately uses it in framing the clauses of the agreement so that he is certain to derive more benefit from the transaction than his less experienced friend, though at the same time he may thoroughly understand that the contract should be drawn up on lines which would ensure that equal benefits would be derived. This he calls business, not theft.

Matthias Alexander

It is quite possible that the thief would scorn to take such advantage of a friend. I have known of such cases; hence the phrase, "Honour among thieves."

Now we do not speak of the other brother as lacking in willpower, but wherein lies the difference in this connection between him and his thief brother?

In the case of the thief, the promise to reform was made. He steals again and again, so that people say in the ordinary way, "He is hopeless, he hasn't the will-power to enable him to reform." As I have before indicated, I fear this is not a correct solution.

For if we admit that in both instances all depends on the point of view, we cannot be surprised that the mere promise to reform is usually futile, and we must furthermore realize that a changed point of view is the royal road to reformation. At the same time, experience of human idiosyncrasies has taught us that the most difficult thing to change is the point of view of subconsciously controlled mankind. The lack of power to reform is the result of the usually partial failure of the subconscious mental mechanisms in a sphere demanding reasoned judgment.

As a matter of fact this man possesses a great amount of willpower and energy in certain directions, just as he probably lacks it in others. This applies equally to his brother and, in a greater or less degree, to every human being. At the same time I think we are justified in concluding that the thief, as compared with his brother, exercises his energy, will-power, and resourcefulness in but limited directions. This applies to all people cursed with what we call criminal tendencies in contrast to their more fortunate fellow-beings. Here we arrive at the point where we are once more confronted with misdirected energies concentrated into narrow channels through abnormal tendencies; hence the over-compensation which inevitably follows.

A thief, unfortunately, too often confines his energies to what to his perverted outlook—the result of a wrong point of view— is a legitimate means of gaining the necessaries of life. From his perverted point of view he merely takes something from another person which he considers he has as much right to possess as any one else, if he is clever enough to get it by any means at his command. I have heard a certain type of Socialist express views which justify this mode of reasoning. His point of view is practically that of the thief, and he needs the same help if he is to come into communication with his reason. We know that men and women have continued to steal for years without being even suspected, and there cannot be any doubt that in thus escaping detection, they prove that they possess forms of exceptional will-power, energy, resourcefulness, courage, determination, and initiative, which, if directed into the right channels, would have made them highly successful and valuable members of society.

It must not be forgotten that if the thief is detected, his punishments are so formidable, not only because of the legal penalties he incurs, but also because of the scorn and derision with which he meets in the social sphere, even among his blood relations, that they would act as a deterrent upon the ordinary person.

Obviously, then, the problem to be solved in connection with the thief or any other criminal, is concerned with the psychophysical conditions which influence him in the direction of crime, and also with the failure of punishment either to change his point of view or to direct his excellent mental and physical gifts into honest and valuable spheres of expression.

We are all aware that a conservative is rarely converted to the liberal viewpoint or vice versa in a day, or a month, or even a year. Such mental changes, in the subconsciously controlled person, should, with rare exceptions, be made gradually and slowly; for the demands of readjustment in the psychophysical self are great, and depend on the conditions present in the particular person. It is conceivable that with certain conditions present, the process of readjustment may bring about such disorganization as may cause a serious crisis. During an experience of this kind the person would for a period be in greater danger than ever,[13] and the length of this period

---

[13] In this connection the following verses (24, 25, 26) from the Gospel according to St. Luke, Chapter XI, are interesting:

24. When the unclean spirit is gone out of a man, he walketh through dry places, seeking rest: and finding none, he saith, I will return unto my house whence I came out.

25. And when he cometh, he findeth it swept and garnished.

26. Then goeth he, and taketh *to him* seven other spirits more wicked than himself; and they enter in, and dwell there: and the last state of

would vary in different people. The process of readjustment in all spheres means immediate interference with the forces of strength and weakness, and in the case of the thief under consideration the force of strength was associated with mental and physical peculiarities in him as evil factors which had more or less controlled him; in fact, they constituted guidance and direction in his case. In all his physical and mental activities, which these evil factors stimulated, he experienced his maximum of confidence and directive power.

Now where his weaknesses were concerned, he had little to depend on. His attempt to reform was a demand for readjustment, which, in turn, meant a period of comparative loss of confidence and directive power. His new efforts needed to be directed into channels where he not only lacked confidence, but where he suffered most from the over-compensation experienced in the past. In reality, his supports were suddenly wrenched from him, and replaced by those which his well-meaning friends and relatives considered infinitely superior and absolutely reliable. Their experiences of life had, to their satisfaction, proved them to be so; but their experiences were not his experiences, their strength was not his strength, their weaknesses were not his weaknesses; and it is in consequence of such facts as these that subconscious control fails, and reasoned conscious control is needed.

If I have succeeded in making my point clear to the reader he will recognize and admit this unfortunate thief's danger. He must, in a way, sympathize with this man who, through no fault of his own, is being directed during the period of comparative helplessness, in a round of unfamiliar and complex experiences by a delusive and debauched subconsciousness. If, on the other hand, conscious reasoned control had been substituted and employed in re-education and co-ordination, the process of readjustment would have presented the minimum of the difficulties and dangers we have enumerated.

In view of the foregoing, are we justified, except in rare instances, in expecting to change the thief any more than the liberal or conservative by ordinary methods on a subconscious basis? The

---

that man is worse than the first.

evidence in the light of experience is against the proposition.

The conservative and the liberal of our example, no less than the thief, are equally dependent on subconscious guidance and control, and are the victims of the particular tendencies, harmful and otherwise, which have developed and become established, as a rule, without recognition, and without any primary appeal to their reasoning faculties.

Therefore, we must turn our attention once more to that psycho-physical process which we call habit, including developments which have their origin in consciousness as well as those which spring from the subconsciousness.

For instance, a man may be, as we say, born a thief. In other words, he is cursed with the subconscious abnormal craving or habit which makes a man a thief by nature.

On the other hand, he may be quite normal at birth, but in early life he may drift into simple and apparently harmless little ways which through carelessness and lack of sound training, develop very slowly and remain unobserved either by the person concerned or by his friends and relatives.

We all know of men and women who became drug fiends merely through wishing to experience the sensation or sensations produced by the drug. In the most unsuspecting way it is repeated at some future time. This innocent beginning has so often developed into the drug habit.

We know of apparently strong-minded scientific men who have taken drugs, in the first instance, from a purely scientific standpoint and so in a seemingly harmless way, but who, in spite of this, have rapidly fallen victims to the drug habit. Exactly the same process has served to create the majority of inebriates.

It is important to keep in mind that different men and different women fall victims to some particular stimulant or drug, whilst they are in absolute mastery of themselves where other seductive influences are concerned.

For instance, A became addicted to a certain drug habit, but although he had taken alcohol from an early age he never became an immoderate drinker. It was not until he came into contact with this particular drug that his latent abnormality or weakness or whatever one chooses to call it became fully manifested. Again, B had lived in China, and had continually smoked opium with the Chinese. He did so for a year without the habit gaining any hold upon him, but the tea habit, on the contrary, became his danger. Despite the fact that his health was seriously affected by over-indulgence in tea, and that according to his medical advisers' opinion he had, by its immoderate use, developed certain troubles which caused him considerable suffering, he continued his excesses in tea-drinking, as others do who come under the influence of drugs, or of alcohol, in one or all of its forms.

When this point is reached these people are, in the words of Emerson, "out of communication with their reason"; a subconscious tendency. Herein lies the explanation of difficulties which they rarely surmount, difficulties which could not remain as such if subconscious control were supplanted by conscious guidance and control of the whole organism; for in practical procedures in life this conscious guidance and control connotes "bringing them once more into communication with their reason" and supplying the "means whereby" of successful readjustment.

That they were out of communication with reason is indicated by the fact that though they knew they were seriously ill, and were told by their doctors that in order to regain health they must abstain from certain foods and drinks, they did not so abstain. Their continuance in indulgence merely satisfied some inward craving which can only become a governing factor as against human reason when men are controlled by the subconscious instead of by the conscious powers; for subconscious control (instinct) is the outcome of experiences in those spheres where the animal senses exercised the great controlling and directing influences in the early stages of man's evolution; whereas conscious control (reasoned experience) through reeducation, co-ordination, and readjustment is the result of the use of the reasoning powers in the conduct of life, by means of which man may fight his abnormal desires for harmful sensory experiences.

The fact that civilized human beings will take wine or sugar or drugs, when conscious that it is gradually undermining health and character, is proof positive of the domination of the physical over the mental self, exactly as in the Stone Age. It shows that in the case of sugar, for instance, they have become victims to the sense of taste. In other words, the sensations produced by the sense of taste influence and finally govern their conduct in this connection, whereas instead they should be governed by the faculties of reason. They have developed vicious complexes in which perverted physical sensations must be satisfied, even at the cost of mental and physical injury, and often of intense pain.

This psycho-physical state does not indicate satisfactory progress on the evolutionary plane up to the present time, and, furthermore, it does not give promise of greater progress in the future under this same subconscious direction. The domination of certain perverted sensations presents another interesting phase, inasmuch as these sensations are very often associated with comparatively superficial complexes.

For instance, take the case of a person who is suffering from the ill effects of taking sugar in harmful quantities. If he happens to decide to abstain from satisfying his taste desires in regard to sugar, and actually abstains for, say, a week or ten days, it often happens that he loses the seductive pleasing sensation formerly derived from sugar, and frequently develops a positive dislike for it.

This also serves to reveal in the majority of people the unreliability of the different senses, such as taste, etc. Of course, in all these cases this unreliability is due to abnormality in one or more directions, usually more, and this fact-emphasizes the absolute necessity for the establishment of those normal conditions which demand conscious guidance and control, for their maintenance in civilization; conditions which tend to eradicate and prevent abnormal cravings and desires in any direction.

When discussing the foregoing phenomena with friends and pupils, I am frequently asked questions like this: "To what are we to attribute the particular manifestations of strength or weakness in different people, where specific abnormal sensations are concerned? "

"Why is one person swayed unduly by some particular sensation which he knows is ruining his health and causing daily suffering, whilst another, equally abnormal and deluded though proof against this failing of his fellow-being, succumbs to some other type of sensory influence?"

It is simply a matter of the psycho-physical make-up of the individual, of his inherent tendencies, and of his general experience of life in different environments. All people whose kinaesthetic systems are debauched and delusive develop some form of perversion or abnormality in sensation. The point of real importance is to eradicate and prevent this kinaesthetic condition in order to make impossible in the human being such domination by sensation.

There is another point which exercises the layman's mind, and that is that great suffering, in consequence of abnormal indulgence in some direction, does not act as a deterrent.

Of course, if these unfortunates were in communication with their reason and were thus consciously guided and controlled, such suffering would serve to prevent them from repeating the experience which caused it.

To those who have studied this curious phase of mental and physical phenomena, it would almost seem that they derived a form of satisfaction or pleasure from such suffering; otherwise, one would conclude, they would not continue to repeat the acts which, in their experience, have been followed by actual pain and discomfort.

And surely there is nothing very unreasonable in this suggestion, seeing that there is little doubt that *ill health* in some people is just as natural as is *health* in others.

It simply means an attempt on the part of nature to do her work where the conditions are *abnormal,* in accordance with the same process as where they are *normal.*

The person enjoying the latter condition abhors suffering and pain, and will act reasonably in order to prevent both, and it is quite consistent with our knowledge and experience of the abnormal in the human organism to incline to the idea that those who are afflicted with abnormal tendencies find a perverted form of pleasure in pain.

And all these suggestions serve to support the theory that the first principle in all training, from the earliest years of child life, must be on a conscious plane of co-ordination, re-education, and readjustment, which will establish a normal kinaesthesia.

The abnormal condition referred to is more or less governed by the senses through the subconsciousness, and we must remember that the great controlling forces in the animal kingdom are chiefly *physical.* It is also in keeping with the purely animal stage of evolution, and any advance from this stage demands that the balance of powers must gradually move in favour of the mental.

The controlling and guiding forces in savage four-footed animals and in the savage black races are practically the same ; and this serves to show that from the evolutionary standpoint the mental progress of these races has not kept pace with their physical evolution from the plane of the savage animal to that of the savage human.

This brings us to the crux of my contentions regarding conscious guidance and control in its widest meaning—that is, as a universal.

Wherever we find the domination of subconscious (instinctive) control, it affords proof that in the lowly evolved states of life the physical is the great controlling force, and we are well aware that this condition does not ensure progress to those higher planes of evolution which should be the goal of civilized growth and development, the goal for which mankind was undoubtedly destined.

The inadequate relative progress of the mental evolution of the black races as compared with that of their physical evolution, when considered in relation to their approximation to the savage animals, cannot be considered other than a most disappointing result. It surely does not furnish any convincing evidence that mankind is likely to advance adequately on the evolutionary plane in civilization by continuing to rely upon the original subconscious guidance and control.

CHAPTER VI - HABITS OF THOUGHT AND OF BODY

"The man who has so far made up his mind about anything that he can no longer reckon freely with that thing, is mad where that thing is concerned."—ALLEN UPWARD, *The New World*.

WHEN speaking of the case of stammering, cited in Chapter IV, I had occasion to note that it was not an easy task to influence X's conscious mind. The point is this: A patient who submits himself for treatment, whether to a medical man or to any other practitioner, may Do what he is told, but will not or cannot THINK as he is told. In ordinary practice the man who has taken a medical degree disregards this mental attitude in ninety-nine cases out of a hundred. Medicine, diet, or exercise is prescribed, and if the patient obediently follows the mechanical directions given with regard to the prescriptions, he is considered a good patient. The doctor does not trouble as to the patient's mode of thinking, except in that one case out of a hundred, possibly a case of flagrant hypochondria.

Indeed, I am willing to maintain and prove in this connection that a very large percentage of cases which are now being treated in our public and private lunatic asylums have been allowed to develop insanity by reason of this disregard of the mental attitude. I cannot stop now to consider this interesting subject of insanity, but I must note in passing that the very large percentage of the cases I have mentioned should never have been allowed to arrive at the condition which made it necessary to send them to an asylum in the first instance. Very many of them, so far from lacking mental control, possess minds of quite exceptional ability. Some are instances of subjects who in the first place have assumed a deliberate attitude to subserve a private end, such as the avoidance of uncongenial work, or the over-indulgence of some desire or perverted sense, the result being that the attitude which was first adopted deliberately became afterwards a fixed habit, and so uncontrollable.

When therefore we are seeking to give a patient conscious control, *the consideration of mental attitude must precede the performance of the act prescribed.* The act performed is of less consequence than the manner of its performance. It is nevertheless a remarkable fact that although the patient or inquirer into the system may apprehend this truth, he often finds an enormous difficulty in altering some trifling habit of thought which stands between him and the benefit he clearly expects. And the simple explanation of this apparently strange enigma is that the majority of people fall into a mechanical habit of thought quite as easily as they fall into the mechanical habit of body which is the immediate consequence.

I will take an instance from a subject outside my own province in order to bring the matter home, but I will preface my illustration by pointing out that I personally am not in the least concerned to alter the habit of thought of either of the persons I bring forward as examples, and I only cite wellknown political propaganda in order to give vividness to my picture.

Let us suppose, then, that A is a convinced Free-trader, and that Z is no less certain of the glorious possibilities of Protection, and let us set A and Z to argue the matter. We notice at once that when A is speaking Z's endeavours are confined to catching him in a misstatement or in a fault of logic, and A's attitude is precisely the same when Z holds the stage. Neither partisan has the least intention from the outset of altering his creed, nor could either be convinced by the facts and arguments of the other, however sound. This is a fact within the experience of every intelligent person. The disputants have so influenced their own minds that they are incapable of receiving certain impressions; a part of their intelligence normally susceptible of receiving new ideas, even if such ideas are opposed to earlier conceptions, is in a state of anaesthesia: it is shut off, put out of action. The habit of mind which has been formed mechanically translates all the arguments of an opponent into misconceptions or fallacies. Neither disputant in our illustration has the least intention or desire to approach the subject with an open mind. Unfortunately, the rigid habit of mind does not only apply to political issues; it is evidenced in all the thoughts and acts of our daily life, and is the cause of many demonstrable evils.

And touching this question of mental rigidity, I may cite a very valuable criticism from Mr. William Archer, the well known London dramatic critic, on the primary point of the "Desirability of the Open Mind." This criticism was published in *The Morning Leader* for 17th December, 1910. I replied in the same paper, and my answer was

Matthias Alexander

published on 23rd December, 1910.

As this brief discussion illustrates very clearly the misconception which most easily arises with regard to this question, I now reprint these two letters, precisely as they originally appeared.

THE OPEN MIND
By William Archer

"In the fifth chapter of an able and interesting book by Mr. Matthias Alexander, entitled *Man's Supreme Inheritance* (Methuen), there occurs a passage which I propose to take as the text of this week's discourse. Treating of ' mechanical habits of thought,' Mr. Alexander says:

"'Let us suppose that A is a convinced Free Trader, and that Z is no less certain of the glorious possibilities of Protection, and let us set A and Z to argue the matter. We notice at once that when A is speaking, Z's endeavours are confined to catching him in a misstatement or in a fault of logic, and A's attitude is precisely the same when Z holds the stage. Neither partisan has the least intention from the outset of altering his creed, nor could either be convinced by the facts and arguments of the other, however sound.... The habit of mind which has been formed mechanically translates all the arguments of an opponent into misconceptions or fallacies. Neither disputant has the least desire to approach the subject with an open mind. Unfortunately this rigid habit of mind does not only apply to the issues of government; it is evidenced in all the thoughts and acts of our daily life, and is the cause of many demonstrable evils.'

Very often, of course, the fact is as Mr. Alexander states it; but can we, I wonder, accept the ideal of the 'open mind' implied in his illustration? Is not a certain stability of conviction absolutely necessary to the efficient conduct of the business of life? And are we not almost as apt to err on the side of impressionability as on the side of rigidity? I seem to remember a warning in Scripture against being ' blown about by every wind of doctrine.'

If we reflect for a moment, I think we shall see that the amount of open-mindedness which reason demands must vary according to the nature of the question at issue. On a question of fact, which is capable of absolute demonstration, it is, of course, folly to let prejudice or bias prevent us from perceiving the truth. But it is not on such questions that disputes commonly arise. Theology, I fancy, is, in the modern world, almost the only influence that frequently leads people to close their minds against demonstrable facts or overwhelming probabilities. But of the most important questions in life, many are not questions of fact at all, while as to others, the evidence is so complex or so inaccessible that demonstration is not, as the saying goes, humanly possible. It is proverbially futile to argue on questions of taste; for enjoyment consists in a relation of the perceiver to the thing perceived which cannot be produced by force of treason or of reasoning. No doubt, in going to ' Salome ' or to the Post-Impressionist Exhibition, we ought to take with us an open mind; that is to say, we ought not to go in a willfully Philistine or frivolous mood. And in discussing them afterwards, we ought to preserve an open mind, in so far that we ought not to make a law of our own limitations, and accuse of folly or insincerity those people who see more in post-Wagnerism and post-Manetism than (perhaps) we do. Yet even here open-mindedness may be carried to excess; for undoubtedly there exists a great deal of affectation and charlatanism in matters of art, and it would be weak credulity to take every Maudle and Postlewaite at his own valuation. 'A popgun remains a popgun,' says Emerson, 'though the ancient and honourable of this world affirm it to be the crack of doom,' and there are innumerable questions of quality and value on which no one who has any mind at all can possibly keep his mind open.

Let us turn now to political questions of the order suggested by Mr. Alexander's illustration. They are not, as a rule, questions of ascertainable fact, but of speculation or conjecture as to the probable results of a given course of action. They are generally very complex questions; the present issue between the two Houses of Parliament is almost unique in its simplicity. And not only is each question complex in itself; it is inextricably interwoven with other questions of similar complexity. Can we reasonably expect or desire, then, that either A or Z, in a single discussion of such a topic as Tariff Reform, should have his whole system of thought revolutionized? When such a conversion occurs (and I suppose it does sometimes occur) ought we to praise the convert's open mind? Ought we not rather to pity his shallow mind, in which the new conviction can scarcely be deeper rooted than the old? A man's political opinions, I take it, if they have any substance and consistency, are, and ought to be, a sort of mosaic set in a cement of fundamental principle. You may alter the pattern by laborious picking and rearranging, but not by a mere push at a single point. Does it follow from this that political discussion is an idle waste of time? Not at all. It forces us to rethink our thoughts, and to keep them consciously and clearly related to fundamental principles. Also it sifts our arguments; in looking out for our opponent's fallacies we not infrequently become aware of our own. Furthermore, a discussion may form part of the long course of thought, or evolution of feeling, whereby a really valid conversion may be ultimately brought about. Though we may think ourselves wholly unmoved by our opponent's reasoning, a subconscious effect may remain, and may in due time manifest itself. Without our realising it, one or two cubes in our mental mosaic may, in fact, have been loosened. A greater result than this, from any single discussion of a complex political question, is scarcely, I think, to be desired. No doubt it is highly desirable that we should at one time or another have brought a perfectly open mind to the study of such a question as Tariff Reform; and this many of us have done. For my own part, I can honestly say that when Mr. Chamberlain first threw the apple of discord into our midst, I so clearly realized the merely traditional and unreasoned character of my Free Trade ideas, that I was biased, if anything, against them, and fully prepared to find them fallacious. The fact that I have not done so may be due to insufficient or unintelligent study, but certainly not to any initial lack of openness of mind.

"Finally, I would note another limitation to the ideal of the open mind. There are certain questions on which we cannot safely keep our minds open, because we know that that way madness lies. I once spent a whole day at Concord, Mass., arguing with a friend who had become a convert to astrology, and was bent on drawing my horoscope. To that I had no objection; but I cannot pretend that my mind was for a moment open to his arguments. Somewhat more difficult is the case of the Bacon-Shakespeare theory: ought we to keep an open mind on that? I am inclined to answer,' No'; for if we once lose grip of the fact that the whole thing is an insanity, we are in danger of being submerged in a swirling torrent of *'folie lucide.'* The origin and psychological conditions of the illusion are perfectly plain. It is, indeed, one of the oddest and most instructive incidents in the history of the human error, and in that sense worthy of study. Poor Bacon has been forced, by no fault of his own, into the position of the Tichborne Claimant of literature, and one cannot but wonder what he would think of the Onslows, Whalleys, and Kenealys, who are pleading what they believe to be his cause. But a really ' open mind ' on the question is, I conceive, a symptom of an exorbitant love of the marvellous and an imperfect hold upon the reality of things. There are subjects on which no mind can remain open without in some degree losing its balance."

THE OPEN MIND
To the Editor of the "Morning Leader"
"Sir—Although Mr. William Archer has rather misapprehended my point of view in his very interesting article, I would not intrude a reply upon you did I not believe that this question is one that lies at the root of so many physical evils, and that it is a question, therefore, which must not be hastily put on one side—as, no doubt, many of your readers will be inclined to put it after their perusal of Mr. Archer's temperate and, apparently, logical reasoning. I say ' apparently,' because, though his syllogism is sound enough, it is based on a faulty premise due to his. misapprehension of my statement; doubtless, I am to blame for not having made myself fully comprehensible.

"In the first place, let me admit at once that the whole question is relative. Mr. Archer's implied example of the man ' blown about by every wind of doctrine' is an example, from my point of view, of rigidity rather than plasticity, inasmuch as he is necessarily a hysterical neurotic, and is almost entirely dependent on his subconscious processes. Now, it is these very subconscious processes which restrict the use of the conscious, reasoning centres; which form what we call habits of mind, that, becoming fixed, are almost beyond the control of reason; which, in extreme cases, take possession of what was once the intelligence, and are manifested as the *idee fixe,* the obsession, the monomaniacal tendency.

But, disregarding these extremes, let me take an example

49

from ordinary life, and perhaps no better one could be offered than Mr. Archer's own of the Bacon-Shakespeare controversy, a subject, among others, which Mr. Archer suggests is sufficient to upset our reason, should we attempt to maintain an open mind with regard to it.

"As a matter of fact, what he conceives as an open mind here is a mind with an inclination to be perverted (or converted) by specious reasoning. The right attitude of the open mind in this case is,' I have weighed the arguments in favour of Bacon's authorship and have found them insufficient, and until such a time as new and better evidence is forthcoming, I shall continue to hold the view I have always held.'

The rigid attitude which I condemn in this connection is the one that says, 'You will never alter my opinion, whatever fresh evidence you may adduce.' In the first example we can come to a conclusion on the evidence; the conscious reason has been exercised and remains in command. It is not until the attitude becomes subconscious and fixed that any danger arises. When that comes about, the man who has decided for Shakespeare's authorship would remain unconvinced in face of any discovery of new evidence. Yet can any one doubt, any one who cares to walk through the world with open eyes as well as an open mind, that the vast majority of opinions given out by the average man and woman have become subconscious habits of thought?

My professional experience has shown me how great an obstacle to the recovery of physical soundness this impeding habit of thought has become. The whole purpose of my book (*Man's Supreme Inheritance*), from which Mr. Archer quotes, is to submit that the course of evolution had tended in the direction of our obtaining conscious control of our own bodies, and argues that this is the only means by which we can rise above the artificial restrictions, often physically poisonous, imposed by civilization. And I assure you, sir, that this ideal of conscious control is absolutely unrealisable by any person who is guided and restrained by these subconscious habits of thought, and who is, in consequence, quite unable to exercise the free use of his intelligence.

So what I intend by the open mind, and in this, I think, Mr.

Archer has not fully understood me, is the just use and exercise of conscious reason, a use which is the rare exception to a very delimiting rule.

Yours, etc.,

"F. MATTHIAS ALEXANDER."

To this letter Mr. Archer did not reply, but this brief correspondence covers very fairly, in my opinion, a statement of the popular objection to the "open mind," and my answer to that objection.

Returning now to my own province of therapeutics, I need hardly give any special instance to carry my point. Of late years much attention has been given to the consideration of mental attitude in relation to disease, and although no clearly defined remedy has been advanced, the condition has been diagnosed and defined. The "fixed idea," hallucination, obsession, are all terms used deliberately to denote a morbid condition, but we have to apply these terms much more widely and grasp the fact that they are applicable to small, disregarded mental habits as well as to the well-defined evils which marked their development. In the case of X, the mental habit which had grown up as the result of postulating, "I can't draw my lip up before speaking," was only another aspect of the attitude of A and Z towards the subject of their discussion, and it was precisely similar in kind. The aggregate of these habits is so characteristic in some cases that we see how easily the fallacy arose of assuming an entity for the subconscious self, a self which at the last analysis is made up of these acquired habits and of certain other habits, some of them labelled instincts, the predisposition to which is our birthright, a predisposition inherited from that long chain of ancestors whose origin goes back to the first dim emergence of active life. Fortunately for us there is not a single one of these habits of mind, with their resultant habits of body, which may not be altered by the inculcation of those principles concerning the true poise of the body which I have called the principles of mechanical advantage,[14] used in co-operation with an understanding of the inhibitory and volitional powers of the

---

[14] Certain aspects of these principles will be found set out in detail in Part II of this volume.

objective mind, by which means these deterrent habits can be raised to conscious control. The false poise and carriage of the body, the incorrect and laboured habits of breathing that are the cause of many troubles besides the obvious ill-effects on the lungs and heart, the degeneration of the muscular system, the partial failure of many vital organs, the morbid fatty conditions that destroy the semblance of men and women to human beings—all these things and many more that combine to cause debility, disease, and death, are the result of incorrect habits of mind and body, all of which may be changed into correct and beneficial habits if once we can clear away that first impeding habit of thought which stands between us and conscious control.

I believe I have at last laid myself quite open to the attack of the habitual objector, a person I am really anxious to conciliate. I have given, him the opportunity of pointing a finger at my last paragraph and saying, "But you only want to change one habit for another! If, as you have implied, the habit of mind is bad, why encourage habits at all, even if they are as you say, 'correct and beneficial'?"

Now this is a point of the first importance. But in the first place it is essential to understand the difference between the habit that is recognized and understood and the habit that is not. The difference in its application to the present case is that the first can be altered at will and the second cannot. For when real conscious control has been obtained, a "habit" need never become fixed. It is not truly a habit at all, but an order or series of orders given to the subordinate controls of the body, which orders will be carried out until countermanded.

It will be understood, therefore, that the word "habit," as generally understood, does not apply to the new discipline which it is my aim to establish in the ordinary subconscious realms of our being. The reasons for this are two:

(1) The conscious, intelligently realized, guiding orders are such as may be continued for all time, becoming more effective year by year until they are established as the real and fundamental guidance and control necessary to that which we understand by the words growth and evolution.

(2) The stimuli to apprehension, or excitement of the fear reflexes, are eliminated by a procedure which teaches the

pupil to take no thought of whether what he calls "practice" is *right or wrong.*

This second statement, however, requires further elucidation; and I feel that a lay description by a pupil of mine may present the case more clearly to the untrained reader than any technical account. The excerpt is from a letter written by the Rev. W. Pennyman, M.A.:

"One great feature of Mr. Alexander's system as seen in practical use is that the individual loses every suggestion of *strain.* He becomes perfectly ,'lissom' in body; all strains and tensions disappear, and his body works like an oiled machine. Moreover, his system has a reflex result, upon the mind of the patient, and a general condition of buoyancy and freedom, and indeed of gaiety of spirit takes the place of the old jaded mental position. It is the pouring in of new wine, but the bottles must also be new or they will burst, and this is exactly what Mr. Alexander's treatment does. It creates the new bottles, and then the new wine can be poured in, freely and fully."

This quotation, however, describes a result, and the means to its achievement can be attained only under certain conditions. There must be, in the first place, a clear realization by the pupil that he suffers from a defect or defects needing eradication. In the second place, the teacher must make a lucid diagnosis of such defects and decide upon the means of dealing with them. In the third place, there must be a satisfactory understanding between teacher and pupil of the present conditions and the means proposed to remedy them.

These three preparatory realizations indicate the real psycho-physical significance of the pupil's mental position. He begins by a definite admission that the subconscious factors by which his psycho-physical organism is being guided are limited and unreliable. He acknowledges, in fact, that he suffers from mental delusions regarding his physical acts and that his sensory appreciation, or kinaesthesis, is defective and misleading; in other words, he realizes that his sense register of the amount of muscular tension needed to accomplish even a simple act of everyday life is faulty and harmful, and his mental conception of such conditions as relaxation and concentration impossible in practical application.

For there can be no doubt that man on the subconscious plane now relies too much on a debauched sense of feeling or of sense-appreciation for the guidance of his psycho-physical mechanism, and that he is gradually becoming more and more overbalanced emotionally, with very harmful and far-reaching results.

The results, indeed, are all too obvious, and yet it must be presumed that the individual has endeavoured to do the *right* and not the *wrong* thing. Does any one set out to catch a train relying on a watch which he knows perfectly well is unreliable? Would any sane person place dependence on the reading of a thermometer that he knows to be defective? No, we must admit not only that there is a failure to register accurately in the sensory appreciation, but also that the fault is unrecorded in the conscious mind. And it is for this reason that the pupil must be given a new and correct guiding and controlling centre, before being asked to perform even the simplest acts in accordance with his own idea and judgment.

Some understanding of these slightly technical and practical details is necessary in order to form a clear idea of what is meant by the simple word "habit," which was the origin of this discussion; but I shall return to a fuller analysis of method in this relation in Part II of this work. What I wish to emphasize in this place is that the evil, disturbing habit which it is necessary to eradicate is in the ordinary experience both permanent and unrecognized. It may in some cases have been originally incurred above the plane of reason, but this form of habit is invariably perpetuated in the subconsciousness. On the other hand, the mode of functioning which is substituted, but which may nevertheless be spoken of quite correctly by the same term of "habit," is as subject to control as the routine of a well organized office. Certain rules are established for the ordinary conduct of business, but the controller of that business must be at liberty to break the rules or to modify them at his discretion. The man who allows an office to take precedence of any other consideration—and I have known instances of such a morbid concession to traditional procedure in business houses—is surely and steadily on the way to commercial failure.

I will now take an illustration of the principle from my own practice. Suppose a patient comes to me who has acquired incorrect respiratory habits, and suppose he is plastic and ready to assimilate new methods, and that after receiving the new guiding orders from me, he soon learns consciously to make a proper use of the muscular mechanism which governs the movements of the breathing apparatus, a word that fitly describes this particular mechanism of the body. Now it would be absurd to suppose that thereafter this person should in his waking moments deliberately apprehend each separate working of his lungs, any more than we should expect the busy manager of affairs constantly to supervise the routine of his well-ordered staff. He has acquired conscious control of that working, it is true, but once that control has been mastered, the actual movements that follow are given in charge of the "subconscious self," although always on the understanding that a counter order may be given at any moment if necessary. Until, however, such counter order is given, if ever it need be given, the working of the lungs is for all intents and purpose subconscious, though it may be elevated to the level of the conscious at any moment. Thus it will be seen that the difference between the new habit and the old is that the old was our master and ruled us, whilst the new is our servant ready to carry out our lightest wish without question, though always working quietly and unobtrusively on our behalf in accordance with the most recent orders given.

Briefly, as I see it, the subconsciousness in this application is only a synonym for that rigid routine we finally refer to as habit, this rigid routine being the stumbling-block to rapid adaptability, to the assimilation of new ideas, to originality. On the other hand, the consciousness is the synonym for mobility of mind, that mobility which the subconscious control checks and impedes, mobility which will obtain for us physical regeneration and a mental outlook that will make possible for us a new and wider enjoyment of those powers which we all possess, but which are so often deliberately stunted or neglected. Consider this point also in its application to the case of John Doe, cited in my second chapter.

If the mental attitude of that individual had been changed, and he had learned to use his muscles consciously; if, instead of automatically performing a set of muscle-tensing exercises, he had devoted himself to apprehending the control and co-ordination of his muscles, he could have carried his knowledge into every act of his life. In his most sedentary occupations he could have been using and exercising his muscular system without resort to any violent contortions, waving of the arms or kicking of the legs, and I cannot but think that he could better have employed the hours spent in this manner by taking a walk in the open air or by occupying himself with some other form of natural exercise. Still, if in his case certain mild forms of exercise at certain times were necessary, such exercises should have employed his mental and physical powers, and through these agencies he should have used his muscular mechanism in such a way that its uses could have been applied to the simplest acts, such as sitting on a stool and writing at a desk. There would then have been no question of what we have termed "civil war" within his body; the whole physical machinery would have been coordinated and adapted to his way of life.

In an earlier paragraph I pointed out that John Doe was suffering from certain mental and physical delusions, and I endeavoured to show how these delusions militated against his recovery of health. Returning to this point now that the correct method has been indicated, I may use his case to give another example of this method. What John Doe lacked was a conscious and proper recognition of the right uses of the parts of his muscular mechanism, since while he still uses such parts wrongly, the performance of physical exercises will only increase the defects. He will, in fact, merely copy some other person in the performance of a particular exercise, copy him in the outward act, while his own consciousness of the act performed and the means and uses of his muscular mechanism will remain unaltered. Therefore before he attempts any form of physical development he must discover, or find some one who can discover for him, what his defects are in the uses indicated. When this has been done he must proceed to inhibit the guiding sensations which cause him to use the mechanism imperfectly; he must apprehend the position of mechanical advantage, and then by using the new correct guiding sensations or orders, he will be able to bring about the proper use of his muscular mechanism with perfect ease. If the mechanical principle employed is a correct one, every movement will be made with a minimum of effort, and he will not be conscious of the slightest tension. In time a recognition will follow of the new and correct use of the mechanism, which use will then become provisionally established and be employed in the acts of everyday life.

For instance, if we decide that a defect must be got rid of or a mode of action changed, and if we proceed in the ordinary way to eradicate it by any direct means, we shall fail invariably, and with reason. For when defects in the poise of the body, in the use of the muscular mechanisms, and in the equilibrium are present in the human being, the condition thus evidenced is the result of an *undue rigidity* of parts of the muscular mechanisms associated with *undue flaccidity* of others. This undue rigidity is always found in those parts of the muscular mechanisms which are forced to perform duties other than those intended by nature, and are consequently ill-adapted for their function.

As Herbert Spencer writes:

"Each faculty acquires fitness for its function by performing its function; and if its function is performed for it by a substituted agency, none of the required adjustment of nature takes place, but the nature becomes deformed to fit the artificial arrangements instead of the natural arrangements."

Unfortunately, all conscious effort exerted in attempts at physical action causes in the great majority of the people of to-day such tension of the muscular system concerned as to lead to exaggeration rather than eradication of the defects already present. Therefore it is essential at the outset of re-education to bring about the relaxation of the unduly rigid parts of the muscular mechanisms in order to secure the correct use of the inadequately employed and wrongly co-ordinated parts.

Let us take for example the case of a man who habitually stiffens his neck in walking, sitting, or other ordinary acts of life. This is a sign that he is endeavouring to do with the muscles of his neck the work which should be performed by certain other muscles of his body, notably those of the back. Now if he is told to relax those stiffened muscles of the neck and obeys the order, this mere act of relaxation deals only with an effect, and does not quicken his consciousness of the use of the right mechanism which he should use in place of those relaxed. The desire to stiffen the neck muscles should be inhibited as a preliminary (which is not the same thing at all as a direct order to relax the muscles themselves), and then the true uses of the muscular mechanism, i.e., the means of placing the body in a position of mechanical advantage, must be studied, when the work will naturally devolve on those muscles intended to carry it out, and the neck will be relaxed unconsciously. In this case the conscious orders, by which I mean the orders given to the right muscles, are preventive orders, and the due sequence of cause and effect is maintained.

I will here note only one more point in concluding my reference to the hypothetical John Doe, who, nevertheless, stands as the representative of a very large body of people. This point is the question of the storing and reserving of energy, and, to use a phrase which has a mechanical equivalent, the registration of tension. If you ask a man to lift a *papiermache* imitation of an enormous dumb-bell, leading him to believe that it is almost beyond his capacity to raise it from the floor, he will exert his full power in the effort to do that which he could perform with the greatest ease. In a lesser degree the same expenditure of unnecessary force is exerted by the vast majority of "physical-culture" students, and by practically every person in the ordinary duties of daily life. The kinaesthetic system has not been taught to register correctly the tension or, in other words, to gauge accurately the amount of muscular effort required to perform certain acts, the expenditure of effort always being in excess of what is required, an excellent instance of the lack of harmony in the untutored organism. This fact may be easily tested by any interested person who will take the trouble to try its application. Ask a friend to lift a chair or any other object of such weight that, while it may be lifted without great difficulty, will in the process make an undoubted call on the muscular energies. You will see at once that your friend will approach the task with a definite preconception as to the amount of physical tension necessary. His mind is exclusively occupied with the question of his own muscular effort, instead of with the purpose in front of him and the best means to undertake it. Before he has even approached it, he will brace or tense the muscles of his arms, back, neck, etc., and when about to perform the act he will place himself in a position which is actually one of mechanical disadvantage as far as he is concerned. Not only are all these preparations of course quite unnecessary, but the whole attitude of mind towards the task is wrong. In such instances as this, any preconception as to the degree of tension required is out of place. If we desire to lift a weight with the least possible waste of energy, we should approach it and grasp it with relaxed muscles, assuming the position of greatest possible mechanical advantage, and then gradually exert our muscular energies until sufficient power is attained to overcome the resistance.

Returning now to the consideration of that bias or predisposing habit of mind which so often balks us at the outset, we may see at once that this predisposition takes many curious forms.

Sometimes it is frankly objective, and is outlined in the statement, "Well, I don't believe in all this, but I may as well try it." In this form a single unlooked-for result is generally enough to change disbelief into credulity. I write the word "credulity" with intention, for I mean to imply that the reaction in a certain type of mind is little, if any, better than the profession of disbelief. What is required is not prejudice in either direction, but a calm, clear, open-eyed intelligence, a ready, adaptive outlook, an outlook, believe me, which does not connote indefiniteness of purpose or uncertainty of initiative. Another form of predisposition arises from lack of purpose, and the mental habits that go with this condition are hard to eradicate, more particularly when the original feebleness has led to some form of hypochondria or nervous disease which has been treated with the usual disregard of the radical evil. It is not difficult for the most superficial inquirer to understand that in treating cases like these any method which relieves the subject still further of the exercise of initiative—such a method as the rest cure, for instance, though I could quote many others— only increases the original evil. The lack of purpose is pandered to and cultivated, and after the six weeks or so of treatment the patient returns to his or her duties in ordinary life even more unfitted than before to perform them. As I have said before no account is taken of the instinct for self-preservation or the will to live. This is the very mainspring of human life, yet in the routine of our protected civilization even its power tends at times to become relaxed, and the machinery runs down.

The machinery should then be wound up again, instead of being allowed to become still further relaxed by resting. This lack of purpose, the immediate effect of our educational methods, is unhappily very common in all classes, but especially among those who have no occupation, or those whose employment is a mechanical routine which does not exercise the powers of initiative. The curious thing about this very large class is that they do not really want to be cured. They may be suffering from many physical disabilities or from actual physical pain, and they may and will protest most earnestly that they want to be free from their pains and disabilities, but in face of the evidence we must admit that if the objective wish is really there, it is so feeble as to be nonexistent for all practical purposes. In many cases this attitude of submission to illness is the outcome of a strong subjective habit. The trouble, whatever it is, is endured in the first instance; it is looked upon as a nuisance, perhaps, but not as an intolerable nuisance; no steps are taken to get rid of it, and the trouble grows until, by degrees, it is looked upon as a necessity. Then at last, when the trouble has increased until it threatens the interruption of all ordinary occupations, the sufferer seeks a remedy. But the habit of submission has grown too strong, and as long as the disease can be kept within certain bounds, no effort is made to fight it. This is of course one of the commonest experiences in the healing profession. A patient is treated and benefited and seems on the high road to perfect health. Then follows a relapse. The first question put is, "Have you been following the treatment?" and the answer, if the patient is truthful, is "I forgot," or "I didn't bother any more about it." In a recent experience of a medical friend of mine, a patient confessed to having stayed in the house for a week after a certain relapse occurred, although the very essence of the prescription by which he had previously benefited was to be in the fresh air as much as possible. This simply means that the subjective habit of submission has grown so strong that the objective mind, weakened in its turn by the neglect of its guiding functions, is unable to conquer it. No prescription or course of treatment can have any effect on such a patient as this, unless the subjective habit can be brought within the sphere of conscious control. In other cases this apparent lack of desire for health is due to an attachment to some dearly loved habit, which must be given up if the proper functions of the body are to be resumed. It may be a habit of petty self-indulgence or one that is imminently threatening the collapse of the vital processes, but the attachment to it is so strong that the enfeebled objective mind prefers to hold to the habit and risk death sooner than make the effort of opposing it. Even in cases where no harm can be traced directly to a markedly influencing habit, the general all-pervading habit of lassitude or inertia is so strong that any regime which may be prescribed is distasteful if it involves, as it must, the exercise of those powers which have been allowed to fall more or less into disuse.

Space will not permit of my giving further instances of the predisposing habit, but very little introspection on the part of my readers should enable them to diagnose their own peculiar mental habits, the first step towards being rid of them. We must always remember that the vast majority of human beings live very narrow lives, doing the same thing and thinking the same thoughts day by day, and it is this very fact that makes it so necessary that we should acquire conscious control of the mental and physical powers as a whole, for we otherwise run the risk of losing that versatility which is such an essential factor in their development.

If, at this point, the reader feels inclined to analyse these habits and to set about a control of them, I will give him one word of preliminary advice, "Beware of so-called concentration."

This advice is so pertinent to the whole principle that it is worth while to elaborate it. Ask any one you know to concentrate his mind on a subject—anything will do—a place, a person, or a thing. If your friend is willing to play the game and earnestly endeavour to concentrate his mind, he will probably knit his forehead, tense his muscles, clench his hands, and either close his eyes or stare fixedly at some point in the room. As a result his mind is very fully occupied with this unusual condition of the body which can be maintained only by repeated orders from the objective mind. In short, your friend, though he may not know it, is not using his mind for the consideration of the subject you have given him to concentrate upon, but for the consideration of an unusual bodily condition which he calls "concentration." This is true also of the attitude of *attention* required for children in schools; it dissociates the brain instead of compacting it. Personally, I do not believe in any concentration that calls for effort. It is the wish, the conscious desire to do a thing or think a thing, which results in adequate performance. Could Spencer have written his *First Principles,* or Darwin his *Descent of Man,* if either had been forced to any rigid narrowing effort in order to keep his mind on the subject in hand? I do not deny that some work can be done under conditions which necessitate such an artificially arduous effort, but I do deny that it is ever the best work. Nor will I admit that such a case as that of Sir Walter Scott can logically be argued against this view. For the real earnest wish to write the Waverley novels was there, even if it originated in the desire to pay the debts he took upon himself, and not in the desire to write the novels because he took a pleasure in the actual performance. Briefly, our application of the word "concentration" denotes a conflict which is a morbid condition and a form of illness; singleness of purpose is quite another thing. If you try to straighten your arm and bend it at the same moment, you may exercise considerable muscular effort, but you will achieve no result, and the analogy applies to the endeavour to delimit the powers of the brain by concentration, and at the same time to exercise them to the full extent. The endeavour represents the conflict of the two postulates "I must" and "I can't"; the fight continues indefinitely, with a constant waste of misapplied effort. Once eradicate the mental habit of thinking that this effort is necessary, once postulate and apprehend the meaning of "I wish" instead of those former contradictions, and what was difficult will become easy, and pleasure will be substituted for pain. We must cultivate, in brief, the deliberate habit of taking up every occupation with the whole mind, with a living desire to carry each action through to a successful accomplishment, a desire which necessitates bringing into play every faculty of the attention. By use this power develops, and it soon becomes as simple to alter a morbid taste which may have been a life-long tendency as to alter the smallest of recently acquired bad habits.

The following is an interesting experience with a pupil who was strongly inclined to a belief in the value and power of concentration. This pupil contested vigorously my attacks on the object of her faith, as practised in accordance with the orthodox conception. She put forward the usual arguments, of course, and I quite failed to make any impression on her mental attitude towards the vexed question under discussion. But at last, some days after our first encounter, my opportunity came. We were not at the time directly discussing concentration, but we were dealing with kindred subjects, and presently my pupil began to speak of the attitudes adopted by people towards the things in life that they like or dislike. Her own plan, she said, with a touch of pride, had been to develop the habit of keeping her mind on other and more pleasant subjects whenever she had been engaged in a task that was unsympathetic to her, and she had so far succeeded in the cultivation of this habit that the disagreeable sensations of any unpleasant duty were no longer experienced by her. I then put one or two questions to her and elucidated among other facts that for years she had been unable "to concentrate" when reading and that this difficulty was becoming constantly more pronounced. Fortunately this instance opened those locked places of her intelligence that I had been unable to reach by argument. I showed her how she had been cultivating a most harmful mental condition, which made concentration on those duties of life which pleased her appear as a necessity. She had been constructing a secret chamber in her mind, as harmful to her general well-being as an undiagnosed tumour might have been to her physical welfare. I am glad to say that she came to admit the truth of my original position and has since begun her efforts to carry out the suggestions I offered for the correction of her bad habit.

And in all such efforts to apprehend and control mental habits, the first and only real difficulty is to overcome the preliminary inertia of mind in order to combat the subjective habit. The brain becomes used to thinking in a certain way, it works in a groove, and when set in action, slides along the familiar, well-worn path; but when once it is lifted out of the groove, it is astonishing how easily it may be directed. At first it will have a tendency to return to its old manner of working by means of one mechanical unintelligent operation, but the groove soon fills, and although thereafter we may be able to use the old path if we choose, we are no longer bound to it.

In concluding this brief note on mental habits I turn my attention particularly to the many who say, "I am quite content as I am." To them I say, firstly, if you are content to be the slave of habits instead of master of your own mind and body, you can never have realized the wonderful inheritance which is yours by right of the fact that you were born a reasoning, intelligent man or woman. But, I say, secondly, and this is of importance to the larger world and is not confined to your intimate circle, "What of the children?" Are you content to rob them of their inheritance, as perhaps you were robbed of yours by your parents? Are you willing to send them out into the world ill-equipped, dependent on precepts and incipient habits, unable to control their own desires, and already well on the way to physical degeneration? Happily, I believe that the means of stirring the inert is being provided. The question of Eugenics, or the science of race culture, is being debated by earnest men and women, and the whole problem of contemporary physical degeneration is one which looms ever larger in the public mind. It is the problem which has exercised me for many years, and which is mainly responsible for the issue of this book, and in my next chapter I shall treat it in connection with the theory of progressive conscious control which I have outlined in the foregoing pages.

CHAPTER VII - RACE CULTURE AND THE TRAINING OF THE CHILDREN

"In what way to treat the body; in what way to treat the mind ; in what way to manage our affairs; in what way to bring up a family; in what way to behave as a citizen; in what way to utilize those sources of happiness which nature supplies,—how to use all our faculties to the greatest advantage; how to live completely? And this, being the great thing needful for us to learn, is, by consequence, the great thing which education has to teach. To prepare us for complete living is the function which education has to discharge."—HERBERT SPENCER, Education.

EVERY child is born into the world with a predisposition to certain habits, and furthermore, the child of to-day is not born with the same development of instinct that was the congenital heritage of its ancestors a hundred or even fifty years ago. Many modern children, for example, are born with recognizable physical disadvantages that are the direct result of the gradually deteriorating respiratory and vital functioning of their forbears. For many months, the period varying with the sex and ability of the individual, the vital processes and movements are for all practical purposes independent of any conscious control, and the human infant remains in this helpless, dependent condition much longer than any other animal.

The habits which the child evidences during this protracted period are those hereditary predispositions which are early developed by circumstance and environment, habits of muscular uses, of vital functioning, and of adaptability.   If it were possible to analyse the tendencies of a child when it is, say, twelve months old, we could soon master the science of heredity which is at present so tentative and uncertain in its deductions, but the child's potentialities lie hidden in the mysterious groupings and arrangement of its cells and tissues, hidden beyond the reach of any analysis. The child is our material; within certain wide limits we may mould it to the shape we desire. But even at birth it is differentiated from other children; our limits may be wide, but they are fixed. Within those limits, however, our capacity for good and evil is very great.

There are two methods by which a child learns. The first and, in earlier years, the predominant method is by imitation; the second is by precept or directly administered instruction, positive or negative.

With regard to the first method, parents of every class will admit the fact not only that children imitate those who are with them during those early plastic years, but that the child's first efforts to adapt itself to the conditions surrounding it are based almost exclusively on imitation. For despite the many thousand years during which some form of civilization has been in existence, no child has yet been born into the world with hereditary instincts tending to fit it for any particular society. Its language and manners, for instance, are modelled entirely on the speech and habits of those who have charge of it. The child descended from a hundred kings will speak the language and adopt the manners of the East End should it be reared among these associations; and the son of an Australian aboriginal would speak the English tongue and with certain limitations behave as a civilized child if brought up with English people.

No one denies this fact; it has been proved and accepted, yet how often do we seek to make a practical application of our knowledge? Although the science of heredity is still tentative and indeterminate, no reasoning person can doubt from this and other instances that in the vast majority of cases at least, the influence of heredity can be practically eradicated. Personally, I see very clearly from facts of my own observation that when the characteristics of the father and mother are analysed, and their faults and virtues understood, a proper training of the children will prevent the same faults and encourage the same virtues in their children.

To appreciate to the utmost the effect of training upon the children, we must remember that the first tastes, likes, or dislikes of the infant begin to be developed during the first two or three days after birth. Long before the infant is a month old, habits, tending to become fixed habits, have been developed, and if these habits are not harmful, well and good. The first sense developed is the sense of taste, a sense that develops very quickly and needs the most careful attention. Artificial feeding is in itself a very serious danger, but when this feeding is in the hands of careless or ignorant persons the danger becomes increased a hundredfold. An instance of this is the common idea that considerable quantities of sugar should be added to the milk.

This is done very often to induce the child to take food against its natural desire. It may be that the child has been suffering from some slight internal derangement, and Nature's remedy has been to affect the child with a distaste for food in order to give the stomach a rest. Then the unthinking mother tempts the child with sugar, and all sorts of internal trouble may follow. But in such a case as this the taste for a particular thing, such as sugar, is encouraged, and apart from the direct harm which may result, the habit becomes the master of the child, and may rule it through life; the child, in fact, is sent out into the world the slave of the sense of taste.

Unfortunately, in ninety cases out of a hundred, children up to the age of six or seven years are allowed to acquire very decided tastes for things which are harmful. Women are not trained for the sphere of motherhood, they do not give these matters the thought and attention they deserve, and hence they do not understand the most elementary principles concerning the future welfare of their offspring in such matters as feeding and sense guidance. Children are not taught to cultivate a taste for wholesome, nourishing foods, but are tempted, and their incipient habits pandered to, by such additions as the sugar I have more particularly cited.

At the present time I know a child of five years old whose taste is already perverted by the method, or lack of method, I have indicated. This child dislikes milk unless undue quantities of sugar are added, will not eat such food as milk puddings or brown bread, and has a strong distaste for cream. It is almost impossible to make the child eat vegetables of any kind, but he is always ready to take large quantities of meat and sweets. The child is already suffering from malnutrition and serious internal derangement. The latter would be greatly improved by small quantities of olive oil taken daily, but it is only with the greatest difficulty that the child can be induced to take it. If he lives with his parents for the next ten years, he will grow into a weak and ailing boy, and will suffer from the worst forms of digestive trouble and imperfect functioning of the internal organs.

Apropos of this point, I remember hearing a question put to my friend, Dr. Clubbe of Sydney, by a London specialist, who asked what, in Dr. Clubbe's opinion, was the primary cause of the derangement of the natural working of a child's muscular mechanism and respiratory system. The answer was given, without hesitation,

"Toxic poisoning as a result of artificial feeding." The logic of this answer will be readily appreciated by the layman, when he considers the interdependence of every part of the system, for in this case the nerve centres connected with the sensory apparatus of the digestive organs control also the respiratory processes. As a consequence, when these centres are dulled in their action as a result of toxic poisoning, there is a loss of activity in the processes of respiration, with consequent maladjustments of those parts of the muscular mechanism more nearly concerned, and so the whole machine is thrown out of gear.

Thus we see that in such instances the mischief begins very early in the life of the child, and it is carried on and exaggerated with every step in its development. Even in babyhood precept and coercion should come into play. Usually when the child cries, little effort is made to discover the cause. Often the child is soothed by being carried up and down the room. It is wonderful how soon the infant begins to associate some rudiments of cause and effect. The child who is unduly pandered to will soon learn to cry whenever it desires to be rocked or dandled, and thus the foundations of pandering to sensation are quickly laid.

But as the child comes to the observant age its habits begin to grow more quickly. We have admitted that a child imitates its parents or nurses in tricks of manner and speech, yet we do not stop to consider that it will also imitate our carriage of the body, our performance of muscular acts, even our very manner of breathing. This faculty for imitation and adaptation is a wonderful force, and one which we have at our command if only we would pause to consider how we may use it in the right way. The vast majority of wrong habits acquired by children result from their imitation of the imperfect models confronting them. But how many parents attempt to put a right model before their children? How many learn to eradicate their own defects of pose and carriage so that they may be better examples to the child? How many in choosing a nurse will take the trouble to select a girl whom they would like their children to imitate? Very, very few. And the reason is simple. In the first place they do not realize the harmful effect of bad example, and, in the second, the great majority of parents have so little perception of truth in this matter that they are incapable of choosing a girl who is a good specimen of humanity, and are sublimely unconscious of their own crookedness and defects.

Children, too, accept their parents' defects as normal and admirable. The boy of twelve or fourteen never dreams, for instance, that his father's protruding stomach is anything but the condition proper to middle-age, and often, doubtless, figures to himself the time when he will arrive at the same condition.

The time will come when such things as these—I refer to the abnormality of the father—will be considered a disgrace.

What, then, can we hope from these parents who are at the present time so unfit, so incapable of teaching their own children the primer of physical life?   And I may note here that this principle has a wider application than that of the nursery; it holds, also, in connection with the model of physical well-being set by the teachers in all primary and secondary schools.

There is no need for me to elaborate this theme. The iniquity of allowing children to be trained in physical exercises, in our Board Schools for instance, by a teacher who is obviously physically unfit, is sufficiently glaring.

The crux of the whole question is that we are progressing towards conscious control, and have not yet realized all that this progress connotes.

Children, as civilization becomes continually more the natural condition, evidence fewer and fewer of their original savage instincts.

In early life they are faced by two evils, if they are developed on the subconscious plane.

If they are trained under the older methods of education they become more and more dependent on their instructors; if under the more recent methods of *"free expression"* (to which I shall presently refer at some length), they are left to the vagaries of the imperfect and inadequate directions of subconscious mechanisms that are the inheritance of a gradually deteriorated psycho-physical functioning of the whole organism.

In such conditions it is not possible for the child to command the kinaesthetic guidance and power essential to satisfactory free expression, or indeed to any other satisfactory form of expression for its latent potentialities. As well expect an automobile, if I may use the simile, to express its capacity when its essential parts have been interfered with in such a way as to misdirect or diminish the right impulses of the machinery. The child of the present day, once it has emerged from its first state of absolute helplessness, and before it has been trained and coerced into certain mental and physical habits, is the most plastic and adaptable of living things. At this stage the complete potentiality of conscious control is present, but can only be developed by the eradication of certain hereditary tendencies or predispositions. Unfortunately, the usual procedure is to thrust certain habits upon it without the least consideration of cause and effect, and to insist upon these habits until they have become subconscious and have passed from the region of intellectual guidance.

I will take one instance as an example of this: the point of right-and-left-handedness. We assume from the outset, and the superstition is so old that its source is untraceable, that a child must learn to depend on its right hand, to the neglect of its left. This superstition has so sunk into our minds by repetition that it has become incorporated in our language. "Dexterous" stands for an admirable, and "sinister" for an inauspicious quality, and we may even find ignorant people at the present day who say that they would never trust a lefthanded person. As a result of this attitude and of the absolute rule laid down that a child must learn to write and use its knife with the right hand only, the number of ambidexterous people is limited to the few who, by some initial accident, used their left hand by preference and were afterwards taught to use their right. In a fairly wide experience I do not remember having heard of a father or mother who has said: "This child may become an artist or a pianist," for example, "and may therefore need to develop the sensitiveness and powers of manipulation of the left hand as well as the right," although I have known of many cases where much time and trouble had to be expended in acquiring the uses of the left hand later in life, such cases as those of persons suffering from writers' cramp and dependent for their living on their ability to use a pen.

I have cited this example of right-handedness because it exhibits the pliability of the physical mechanism in early life, and the manner in which we thoughtlessly bind it to some method of working, without ever stopping to think whether that method is good in itself, or whether it is the one adapted for the conditions of life into which the child will grow. We thrust a rigid rule of physical life and mental outlook upon the children. We are not convinced that the rule is the best, or even that it is a good rule. Often we know, or would know if we gave the matter a moment's consideration, that in our own bodies the rule has not worked particularly well, but it is the rule which was taught to us, and we pass it on either by precept, or by holding up our imperfections for imitation, and then we wonder what is the cause of the prevailing physical degeneration!

What is intended by these methods of education is to inculcate the accumulated and inferentially correct lessons derived from past experience. It is true that the lesson varies according to the religious, political, and social colour of the parent and teacher, but speaking generally, the intention would be logical enough if we could make the primary assumption that each generation starts from the same point—the assumption, in other words, that a baby is born with the same potentialities, the same mental abilities, and assuredly the same physical organism whether he be born in the sixteenth or the twentieth century.

And even as recently as a hundred years ago, that assumption might have been made with some show of reason. For the changes were so slight and have evolved so slowly as to attract little attention. Granted similar conditions of parentage and upbringing, the differences between the child of A.D. 1800 and that of A.D. 1700 were hardly noticeable.

That statement, however, does not apply to the child of 1917. For many years past there has been unrest and dissatisfaction in the world of education. New methods have been tried, superimposed for the most part on the top of the older ones, and even more daring experiments have been made, experiments which sought to throw over the old traditions, bag and baggage. All these trials have so far failed, in my opinion; and one reason for the failure has been due to the fact that educationalists as a body have been unable to recognize the obvious truth that the child of the twentieth century cannot be judged by the old standards.

This truth is so evident to me that I hesitate at the necessity to prove it. It seems incredible to me that any one of my generation could fail to realize the extraordinary difference between the contemporaries of his own growth and the children of our present civilization. I could produce a dozen instances of this difference, but one must suffice in this place. It is, however, an example that is peculiarly typical. For I remember, and my experience has not been in any way an abnormal one, the facility with which the children of my generation learnt the uses of common tools. In a sense they may be said to have inherited a certain dexterity in the handling of such things as a hammer, knife, or saw. To-day many parents are greatly impressed if a child of from two-and-a-half to six years old can use one of these implements with a reasonable show of efficiency. I have known fathers and mothers representative of the average parent to-day who find any instance of this efficiency in their own children an almost startling thing, and certainly matter for boast to their relations and friends.

Unhappily the real difference goes far deeper than this superficial effect would at first seem to indicate. The early attempts of the modern child to employ his physical endowment in such common and necessary acts as walking, running, sitting, or speaking, are far below the standard of ability that I remember a generation ago. The standard of kinaesthetic potentiality has been lowered. Elements that I will not attempt to trace, lest I be tempted on to the fascinating ground of evolutionary theory, have intervened most amazingly in the past thirty years, and the most evident result of this intervention has been the marked change in the subconscious efficiency of the modern child.

Thus, even from the birth of the infant, our problem is not precisely that of the old educationalists; and this primary congenital difference between the children of two generations has been, and is being, exaggerated in the nurseries of the independent classes both in England and America. (Doubtless in other countries of Europe the same effects are being produced, but I prefer to speak only of that which I have observed and closely studied for myself.) There is still a tendency to take all responsibility and initiative away from the child of wealthy parents. Nurses first and governesses later perform every possible act of service that shall relieve the child of trouble. It is not even allowed to invent its own games. Toys are supplied in endless quantities—expensive, ingenious toys, that need no imaginative act to transform them into reduced models of the motors, trains, or animals they are manufactured to represent, and some one, some adult, is always at hand to amuse the child and teach him how to play. I must italicize the absurdity of that last sentence. For what does this teaching

Race Culture and the Training of the Children mean, if it does not mean that it is seeking to substitute the. adult idea of play for the childish one?

In my day, any old brick played the part of a train or a horse, and in the mental act required to see the reality under so uncompromising a guise my imagination was exercised.

Then I, and the other children of my time, grew dissatisfied with so poor a substitute, and as we progressed in experience, the stimulated imaginations found expression in *inventing* and in *making* better replicas of the realities of our childish experience.

And we grew with the exercise.

We had our little responsibilities and we taught ourselves not only how to play but how presently to adapt our play to the great business of social life.

But what equipment is furnished to the child who never has an independent moment throughout its nursery career?

How can such a child hope to succeed in life, should the fortune it hopes to inherit from its parents be suddenly lost or diverted?

Every one knows the answer.

We can see the results in any great city of modern civilization, in London slums and in the Bowery of New York. A few generations of such teaching as this and, we should have had a differentiated race as helpless as the slave-keeping ants.

But although this petrifying method of teaching and supervision is still practised, the reaction against it has already set in both in England and America. Unhappily that reaction has been too violent, as such reactions commonly are. From one extreme of permitting the child no opportunity of the exercise of independent thought and action, we have flown to the other in adopting the principle which is now known as "Free Expression"—a principle which I can show to be no less harmful than over-supervision. In fact, so far as the physical expression of a child is concerned, the methods of Free Expression are even more dangerous than those of the opposite school.

In England, this movement towards "Free Expression" has not so far been crystallized into a definite propaganda, nevertheless a number of thoughtful but unhappily inexpert parents are trying to adopt the principle in their own homes. Mr. Shaw's Preface to his *Misalliance* puts the theory of the method in a very clear and convincing, argument. His main assumption is as follows: "What is a child? An experiment. A fresh attempt to produce the first man made perfect; that is, to make humanity divine. And you will vitiate the experiment if you make the slightest attempt to abort it into some fancy figure of our own...." That represents, of course, an idealist attitude, and every idealistically minded parent in Great Britain who reads that Preface of Mr. Shaw's on "Parents and Children" at once attempts to put the theory into practice. The results, if the theory is persisted in, will be disastrous; and although in many cases the parents realize their error by practical experience before the child reaches the age of seven or so, certain cases I have seen demonstrate all too clearly that much mischief is being done even at the age of seven; faults and bad habits have become so far established that it is sometimes very hard to eradicate them.

And in America the mischief is going farther still. Socalled "free" schools have been instituted which, although they may differ in the detail of their methods, are based on the same underlying principles. As far as I have examined the theory and practice of these schools their purposes are:

(1) To free the child as far as possible from outside interference and restraint.
(2) To place him in the right environment and then to give him materials and allow him activities through which he may "freely express himself."

Now this presupposes, firstly, that the child if left to himself has the power of expressing himself adequately and freely; secondly, that through this expression he can educate himself. How far both these suppositions are fallacies will be understood by any one who has followed my argument and my citations of actual cases even up to this point; but the matter is so important that I do not hesitate to bring forward further evidence to establish my objection to this new and dangerous method.

I will begin by drawing attention to the practical side of two of the channels for self-expression, which are specially insisted upon in schools where the new mode is being practised, namely; dancing and drawing. A friend of mine always refers to them as the two D's, a phrase that refers very explicitly to these two forms of damnation when employed as fundamentals in education.

The method of the "Free Expressionist" is to associate music with the first of these arts. Now music and dancing are, as every one knows, excitements which make a stronger emotional appeal to the primitive than to the more highly evolved races. No drunken man in our civilization ever reaches the stage of anaesthesia and complete loss of self-control attained by the savage under the influence of these two stimuli. But in the schools where I have witnessed children's performances, I have seen the first beginnings of that madness which is the savage's ecstasy. Music in this connection is an artificial stimulus and a very potent one. And though artificial stimuli may be permissible in certain forms of pleasure sought by the reasoning, trained adult, they are uncommonly dangerous incitements to use in the education of a child of six.

Need I defend still further my description of music as an artificial and powerful stimulus? During the war it was reported that the influence of alcohol and drugs had been resorted to by the Germans to drive their men to the attack. But we know that in earlier wars the greatest effects could be attained by music, effects that drive the fighters into the most delirious excesses of savagery. And, doubtless, if the sound of music could have made itself heard above the awful din of guns that precede a modern advance, the old stimulus would have been preferred by the Germans to the administration of drugs. As it is, I have heard that bands are used whenever possible. Full-grown men and women will admit that they can become "drunk" with music, and by "drunk" I mean that the motions of the subconsciousness are excited to such a pitch that they take control, until they completely dominate the reasoning faculties. Alcohol produces this result by partial paralysis of the peripheral cilia, music and dancing by overexaltation of the whole kinaesthetic system. In the latter case, however, no evil effects can be produced in the first instance, without the reasoning consent or submission of the subject. Savages and *young children have not yet learnt to withhold that consent.*

And altogether apart from this question of intoxication — to which by the the way every individual is not susceptible—these unrestrained, unguided efforts of the children to dance are likely to prove extremely harmful. I have watched while first one air and then another has been played on the piano, the intention of these changes being to convey a different form of stimulus with each air, and I admit that the children responded in accordance with the more or less limited kinaesthetic powers at their command. But it was very obvious to me that all these little dancers were more or less imperfectly co-ordinated; that the idea projected from the ideomotor centre constantly missed its proper direction; that subconscious efforts were being made that caused little necks to take up the work that should have been done by little backs; that the larynx was being harmfully depressed in the efforts to breathe adequately, causing both inspiration and expiration to be made through the open mouth instead of through the nostrils; and that the young and still pliable spines were being gradually curved backwards and the stature shortened when the very opposite condition was essential even to a satisfying aesthetic result.

And when we realize that the teachers who witness these lessons are entirely ignorant of the ideal physical conditions that are proper to children, and so are woefully unaware of the dangerous defects that are being initiated by these efforts to dance, we must admit that, as practised, this particular form of free expression is being encouraged at a cost that far outweighs any imagined advantage.

Here, for instance, is an example that came directly under my notice. A little girl six years old was brought to me for kinaesthetic examination, and I found her to be in really excellent physical condition. She was then sent to school, where she became interested in dancing. The dancing at this school was considered a form of free expression, and the children were encouraged to make their own movements, undirected. Different airs were played to which the child was expected to react, and the little girl of my example found great pleasure in this part of her school work and gave much of her time to it, until she was considered to express herself more freely than any of the other children in the form of art she had chosen. I may point out that one of the essential principles of these free-expression schools is to permit a child to choose its own activity and to pursue it for practically as long as it desires.

Her mother, however, became dissatisfied after a time with her child's general condition. Curious and somewhat alarming physical distortions were beginning to manifest themselves, most noticeably a tendency to carry her head on one side, a tendency she was unable to rectify. At last the mother brought back the child to me for re-examination.

Now less than a year before I had passed this child as an unusually fine example of correct physical co-ordination. When she came back to me she was in little better condition than a congenital degenerate. All that fluent co-ordination of her muscular mechanisms had disappeared, and in place of it I found rigid tendons, stiffened muscles, and, worst of all, faulty habits of guidance and control, among them a habit of governing the muscles of her body and legs by stiffening the unrelated muscles of her neck. (Incidentally I may note in passing that in the human being the neck is very often the indicator of inadequate and false controls. There are good reasons why this should be the case, *a priori,* but they are too technical for this book.) A further particular defect was due to a tensing and shortening of the upper muscles of the thighs where they are attached to the torso, a defect that was tending to warp and shorten the child's stature. Lastly—the most significant change of all—the child who a year before had been outspoken and fearless and clear of speech, was now timid and shy, and mumbled her words so badly that I could with difficulty understand her.

Here, then, is a case of a child, starting in the best physical condition, who was placed in what was considered the right environment and permitted the exercise of free activity. And I claim that the harmful result was so inevitable that any one of real experience might have anticipated it with almost absolute certainty.

The second ominous "D" is drawing, and this comes into another category of damnation, since mental rather than physical effects are concerned, although the latter are involved both in the harmful, uncorrected poses adopted by the children when seated at the table, and in the false directions of the ideomotor centres of which only a few reach the essential fingers that are holding, or more often grotesquely clutching, the pencil. It may seem a small thing to the layman that a child should try to guide a pencil by movements of its tongue, but to the expert that confusion of functions is indicative of endless subconscious troubles.

Let me describe the practical procedure of a certain type of "free-drawing" lesson. Pencils, paper, and the usual paraphernalia are placed on tables or desks in different parts of the schoolroom, in the hope

Matthias Alexander

that the child may be tempted to use them in drawing. Then, one day, a pupil takes up a pencil and makes an attempt to draw, another follows his example and so on, until all the pupils have made some kind of effort in this direction.

Now the act of drawing is in the last analysis a mechanical process that concerns the management of the fingers, and the co-ordination of the muscles of the hand and forearm in response to certain visual images conceived in the brain and imaginatively projected on to the paper. And the standard of functioning of the human fingers and hand in this connection depends entirely on the degree of kinaesthetic development of the arm, torso, and joints; in fact on the standard of coordination of the whole organism. It is not surprising, therefore, that hardly one of these more or less defectively coordinated children should have any idea of how to hold a pencil in such a way as will command the freedom, power, and control that will enable him to do himself justice as a draughtsman.

Any attentive and thoughtful observer who will watch the movement and position of these children's fingers, hand, wrist, arm, neck, and body generally, during the varying attempts to draw straight or crooked lines, cannot fail to note the lack of co-ordination between these parts. The fingers are probably attempting to perform the duties of the arm, the shoulders are humped, the head twisted on one side. In short, energies are being projected to parts of the bodily mechanism which have little or no influence on the performance of the desired act of drawing, and the mere waste projection of such energies alone is almost sufficient to nullify the purpose in view.

But I have already said enough to prove that no free expression can come by this means. The right impulse may be in the child's mind, but he has not the physical ability to express it. Not one modern child in ten thousand is born with the gift to draw as we say "by the light of Nature," and that one exceptional child will have his task made easier if he is wisely guided in his first attempts.

But my chief objection to this teaching of drawing is the encouragement it gives to profitless dreaming. Drawing is an art, and we know some of the characteristics that are commonly imputed to the artist—though many of the greatest artists have been exemplarily free from them. These characteristics are eccentricity, lack of balance, power of self-hypnotism, and a general irrationality. Yet surely it cannot be emphasized too strongly that the artist succeeds in spite of these impediments to expression, and not because of them. These characteristics that I have instanced are by-products of the artistic genius. They are developed through erroneous conceptions and overconcentration on a particular creative activity, and time and again in the history of the world these by-products have ruined, incapacitated, and disgraced men of real genius.

Nevertheless, if I can judge by my experience of this form of free expression, the child is encouraged to practise the eccentricity as a means to obtain the gift of drawing, which as a principle is about the same as trying to breed race-horses with weak lungs because it has been noted that certain very fast horses have been rather deficient in this respect. To encourage eccentricity is not to breed genius, and genius itself is more free and more creative when it is not hampered by eccentricity. Let us, at least, have some appreciation of rational cause and effect.

So much for my two "D's," but my general criticism of the "free expression" experiment does not end there. For I must confess that I have been shocked to witness the work that has been going on in these schools. I have seen children of various ages amusing themselves—somewhat inadequately in quite a number of cases—by drawing, dancing, carpentering, and so on, but in hardly a single instance have I seen an example of one of these children employing his physical mechanisms in a correct or *natural* way. I insist upon the use of the word *natural* even though it be applied to such relatively artificial activities as drawing and carpentering. For there is a right, that is to say a most effective, way of holding and using a pencil or a carpenter's tool. But the children I saw commonly sat or stood in positions of the worst mechanical advantage, and the manner in which they held their pencils or their tools demonstrated very clearly that until their management of such instruments was corrected, they could never hope to produce anything but the most clumsy results. Worse still, these children were forming physical habits which would develop in a large majority of cases into positive physical ills. A child who tries to guide its pencil by futile movements of its head, tongue, and shoulders may be preparing the way to ills so farreaching that their origin is often lost sight of.

As an instance of this, I recently had a case of a boy of three-

and-a-half years who suffered from fear reflexes. If a stranger entered a room when the child was present, he would cry and cling to his mother or nurse. At the seaside, after asking to be allowed to bathe with other children, he was subsequently afraid to go near the water. And in many other ways he exhibited unreasoning terrors which, according to the general diagnosis common in such cases, were presumed to be the cause of his general backwardness, a symptom particularly marked in his speech, for he was only able to articulate a few words, and those very imperfectly.

My first examination of him revealed the fact that he lacked proper control of his lips and tongue, and of one internal physical function, the latter chiefly at night. And that the lack of control in these particulars was the direct cause of his psycho-physical condition was very conclusively proved by my treatment of him. Treated on a basis of conscious guidance and control, re-educated and co-ordinated, the child made a rapid advancement, and he progressed towards a condition approximating more closely to what one might call normal, than he had experienced since birth. The fear reflexes became less and less subject to excitement, he grew less irritable, his temper was more controlled, and his outbursts of crying were exhibited far less often.

I have cited this instance to show what strange psychic effects may spring from apparently purely physical causes—though, indeed, the complement of psycho-physical is so unified that it is impossible to divide the components and place them on one plane or the other. In this boy's case the primary cause of the trouble was probably congenital, but equal and greater troubles may arise from much smaller original defects if the initial habit is confirmed and crystallized by use, as I fear will be the case if the child is left to develop itself on the lines of the free expression advocates. It is quite certain, for example, in the case just referred to, that no amount of "free" activity could have released the child from his constrictions whilst the influence caused by his malco-ordinations still existed.

But surely I have given evidence enough to prove my case against this last development in education. In an ideal world into which children were born with ideal capacities, Mr. Shaw's thesis might have some weight. In this rapidly changing world of the twentieth century we require, more than ever before, a system that shall guide and direct the child during his earlier years. This implies no contradiction of what I have said earlier anent the method of constant supervision. The necessary correction of physical and mental faults that I am advocating is a very different thing from the attempt to mould a child into one particular preconceived form. I would only insist that the children of to-day, born as they are with very feeble powers of instinctive control, absolutely require certain definite instructions by which to guide themselves before they can be left to free activity. And these directions must be based on a principle that will help the child to employ his various mechanisms to the best advantage in his daily activities. These directions involve no interference with what the child has to express; they represent merely a cultivation and development of the *means* whereby he may find adequate and satisfying release for his potentialities.

It is true that the foregoing principles must and will involve certain necessary prohibitions, but if we select those essentials that deal with the root cause of the evil instead of with the effects, we render unnecessary the continual admonitions and "naggings" which represented one of the vices of the old system, a vice from which it has been the object of the new education to free the child.

To sum up this aspect of child-training, I find that on the whole the methods of the older educationalists, with their definite prohibitions and their exact instructions, were less harmful than the extremes of the modern school that would base their schemes of education upon a child's instinctive reactions. The older methods failed, I admit, for one reason, because the system was carried too far; for another, because the injunctions and prohibitions were based on tradition, prejudice, and ignorance, instead of upon a scientific principle dictated by reason. But the new methods fail because they are founded on an entirely erroneous assumption which is demonstrably fallacious. Can any method be defended that is open to such a charge?

Give a child conscious control and you give him poise, the essential starting-point for education. Without that poise, which is a result aimed at by neither the old nor the new methods of education, he will presently be cramped and distorted by his environment. For although you may choose the environment of a nursery or a school, there are few indeed who can choose their desired environment in the world at large. But give the child poise and the reasoned control of his physical being, and you fit him for any and every mode of life; he will have wonderful powers of adapting himself to any and every environment that may surround him. And if he be one of those exceptional individuals who, by some rare gift of nature or by some force of personality, are able to bend life to their own needs, be very sure that, so far from having suppressed his power of free expression, you will have strengthened and perfected just those abilities which will enable the genius to put forth all that is best and greatest in him.

My last charge against the advocates of free expression is that they themselves are not free. So many propagandists and teachers show an unwarranted intolerance towards the exponents of the old systems. They are, in fact, too constricted in their mental attitude to give play to their imagination. From one extreme they have flown to the other, and so have missed the way of the great middle course which is wide enough to accommodate all shades of opinion.

For let me state clearly, in concluding this comment on a new method, that I am, myself, a strong advocate for free expression, rightly understood. But I am convinced by long observation and experiment that the untrained child has not the adequate power of free expression. There are certain mechanical and other laws, deduced from untold centuries of human experience, laws that are only in the rarest cases unconsciously followed by the natural child of to-day. (One of these rare cases that has recently come under my notice has been the billiard-playing of Mr. George Gray. I am of the opinion that the mechanical principle of the position adopted by him could be scientifically demonstrated as being as nearly perfect for its particular purpose as any position could be. And according to my observation of him, Mr. Gray manifests in his play the most remarkable and controlled kinaesthetic development I have yet witnessed. But how many George Grays has the world so far produced?)

Over twenty-two years ago in Australia, I was teaching what I still believe to be the true meaning of free expression. My pupils in this case came to me for lessons in vocal and dramatic expression. Now by the old methods these pupils would have been taught to imitate their master very accurately in vocal and facial expression, in gesture, in the manner of voice production; and it would have been at once apparent to any one acquainted with the manner and methods of the teachers, where each pupil had received his training. Furthermore, pupils educated by those methods were taught to interpret each poem, scene, or passage on the exact lines that were considered correct by their respective teachers.

My own method, which at that time was regarded as very radical and subversive, was to give my pupils certain lessons in re-education and co-ordination on a basis of conscious guidance and control, and in this way I gave the reciter, actor, or potential artist the means of employing to the best advantage his powers of vocal, facial, and dramatic expression, gesture, etc. He could then safely be permitted to develop his own characteristics. A few suggestions might be necessary as to interpretation, but the individual manner was his own. No pupil of mine could be pointed to as representing some narrow school of expression, although most of them could be recognized by the confidence and freedom of their performances.

And in this connection it may be of interest to my readers to know that in 1902-3 I decided to test the principles I advocated, and to this end I organized performances of "Hamlet" and "The Merchant of Venice," for which I gave special training on the lines I have just indicated to young men and women, none of whom had previously appeared in a public performance of any kind whatsoever. I trained all these young people on the principles of conscious guidance and control, principles that I had then developed and practised. My friends and critics naturally anticipated a wonderful exhibition of "stage fright" on the evening of the first performance, but as a matter of fact not one of my young students had the least apprehension of that terror. By the time they were ready to appear the idea of "stage fright" was one that seemed to them the merest absurdity. It may be said that they did not understand what was meant by such a condition. And this, although I would not allow a prompter on the nights of the public performance! I regard this as one of the most convincing public demonstrations I have yet made of the wonderful command and selfpossession that may be attained by the inculcation of these principles. For it must be observed that I sent these tyros to the performance capable of expressing their own individualities.

If they had been hedged about or boxed in by an endless series of "Dont's" confining their performances by a rigid set of rules, the majority of them would almost certainly have broken down within the first two minutes.

On the other hand, it is hardly necessary to picture the chaos that would have ensued had I sent them on the stage without training of any kind, poor, helpless, ignorant examples of what they supposed to be free expression. The foregoing is an example of education in only one sphere of art, but it serves as an excellent indication of the essential needs of education, in general, where the child is concerned. We must give the child of to-day and of the future, as a fundamental of education, as complete a command of his or her kinaesthetic systems as is possible, so that the highest possible standard of "free expression" may be given in every sphere of life and in all forms of human activity.

We must build up, co-ordinate, and readjust the human machine so that it may be *in tune*.

We are all acquainted with the expression *"tune up"* where the automobile is concerned, and when we wish to command the best expression of this machine we avail ourselves of the *"tuning-up"* process of the mechanical expert.

And as the human organism is, as Huxley says, a machine, we must remember that if we wish it to express its potentialities adequately it must be *"in tune."*

This will represent what we consider to be that satisfactory condition of the child's kinaesthetic systems which will enable him to express himself freely and adequately.

It constitutes the "means whereby" of free and full expression, of adaptability to the ever-changing environment of civilized life, and to all that these two essentials connote.

In this note on race culture and the training of children, I have thus far dwelt almost exclusively on the earlier years of childhood. But I have much to say at some future time of the questions of primary and secondary education—that is, of the boy and girl at school between the ages of, say, seven and eighteen. No one who has read so far with attention and has earnestly attempted to comprehend my point of view, will now be able to urge that the question of education, secular or religious; is outside my province, for the mental and physical are so inextricably combined that we cannot consider the one without the other, but, at the risk of being accused of repetition,

I will briefly state my case in this connection once again, as follows:

I wish to postulate:

That conscious guidance and control, as a universal, must be the fundamental of future education.

That civilization and education, as manifested up to the present, cannot be said to have compelled man to advance adequately from the lower to those higher planes of satisfactory evolution, where his savage animal instincts will not in any circumstances, or in response to any stimuli, dominate his transcendent tendencies, or put him out of communication with his reason.

That mankind should progress by slow continuous processes from one stage of evolution to another.

This will be particularly the case when he is passing from his animal subconscious stage to the higher, reasoned conscious stages, during which process he will develop a new subconsciousness (cultivated, not inherited) under the guidance of consciousness, likewise an increasing control which holds his animal proclivities in check. That the evolutionary progress from childhood to adolescence, and so through the vicissitudes of life which follow, is determined by the process adopted, the ratio of progress being in accordance with the standard of efficacy of this process, and that this principle of evolution applies equally to a nation.

That subconsciously developed mechanisms (subconscious guidance and control) function satisfactorily during those stages of our evolution which approximate to the more or less animal plane.

That the old moderate methods of education are not incompatible with cultivation and development on the animal subconscious plane.

That "free expression" principles cannot bring satisfactory results while the subject's mechanisms are operated by inherited subconscious guidance and control.

For this very reason, all aid to progressive development must conform to the principle of the projection of guiding orders and controls in the right direction or directions with the simultaneous employment of positions of mechanical advantage, irrespective of the correctness or otherwise of the immediate result. The result may be unsatisfactory to-day and tomorrow, or during the next week, but if the position of mechanical advantage is employed and orders and controls in the right direction are held in mind and projected again and again, a new and correct complex sooner or later supersedes the old vicious one, and becomes permanently established.

That consciously controlled mechanisms (conscious guidance and control) are essential to man's satisfactory development and progress to the higher stages of his evolution; and to that continued adequate vital functioning of his physical or mental organism necessary in these advanced stages, where more rapid adaptability to the swiftly and ever-changing environment, and the power to *see* and *comprehend new ideas,* are the urgent demands of an advancing civilization.

That consciously controlled mechanisms are essential to the successful inculcation of the principle of "free expression" and all that it connotes in Education.

Conscious guidance and control, as the fundamental in education, commands the fundamentals of "free expression." The words free or freedom are herein used in their true meaning, not in the ordinary acceptation. I refer to the point of view which causes one to ask, " Is there such a thing as real freedom?" For we know that we cannot have freedom without restraint, any more than we can have psycho-physical harmony without antagonism.

It is said that the dividing line between tragedy and comedy is not one that the majority of people readily recognize, and this is also the case in regard to what is called freedom and licence. This is the danger which the new democracies of the world are facing at this very moment, and their dangers will be increased a thousandfold in the near future, when they will be called upon to pass through that critical period of readjustment which must follow the present world crisis.

In this matter of education I am, admittedly, an iconoclast. I would fain break down the idols of tradition and set up new concepts. In no matters do we see more plainly the harmful effect of the rigid convention than in this matter of teaching. We speak commonly of training the minds of children. It is a happy expression in its origin, and we still retain its proper intention when we apply the word to its uses in horticulture.

The gardener does, indeed, train the young growth. He draws it out to the light and warmth and leads it into the conditions most helpful for its development. And so, in teaching, the first essential should be to cultivate the uses of the mind and body, and not, as is so often the case, to neglect the instrument of thought and reason by the inculcation of fixed rules which have never been examined.

Again, where ideas that are patently erroneous have already been formed in the child's mind, the teacher should take pains to apprehend these preconceptions, and in dealing with them he should not attempt to overlay them, but should eradicate them as far as possible before teaching or submitting the new and correct idea.

I say "teaching or submitting," and perhaps the latter word better expresses my meaning, for by teaching understand the placing of facts, for and against, before the child in such a way as to appeal to his reasoning faculties, and to his latent powers of originality.   He should be allowed to think for himself, and should not be crammed with other people's ideas, or one side only of a controversial subject.

Why should not the child's powers of intelligence be trained?

Why should they be stunted by our forcing him to accept the preconceived ideas and traditions which have been handed down from generation to generation, without examination, without reason, *without inquiry as to their truth or origin?* The human mind of to-day is suffering from partial paralysis by this method of forcing these unreasoned and antiquated principles upon the young and plastic intelligence.

The educational system itself is grievously inadequate and detrimental, as all thinking educationalists are aware, but the decision regarding the necessity for physical exercise and "deep breathing" in our schools has added another evil. I wish to say here deliberately that the many systems of physical training generally adopted show an almost criminal neglect of rational method, and of the test which can demonstrably prove the practice to be unsound and hurtful.

Some years ago I wrote in the *Pall Mall Gazette:*

"I will merely point out that in our schools and in the Army human beings are actually being developed into deformities by breathing and physical exercises'. I have before me a book on the breathing exercises which are used in the Army, and any person reasonably versed in physiology and psychology, and knowing they are inseparable in practice, will at once understand why so much harm. results from them. Take either the officers or the men. In a greater or less degree the unduly protruded upper chests (development of emphysema), unduly hollowed backs (lordosis), stiff necks, rigid thorax, and other physical eccentricities have been cultivated. It is for these reasons that heart troubles, varicose veins, emphysema, and mouth breathing (in exercise) are so much in evidence in the Army. As this is a matter of *national importance, I am prepared to give the time necessary to prove to the authorities (medical or official) connected with the Army, the schools, or the sanatoria, that the ' deep breathing' and physical exercises in vogue are doing far more harm than good,* and are laying the foundations of much graver trouble in the future. The truth is that all exercises involving ' deep breathing ' cause an exaggeration of the defective muscular co-ordination already present, so that even if one bad habit is eradicated, many others— often more harmful— are cultivated."

And again in my pamphlet *Why We Breathe Incorrectly* (Nov. 1909) I wrote:

"Let me make myself clear by explaining that the man who breathes incorrectly and inadequately, does so as an immediate and inevitable consequence of abnormal and harmful conditions of certain parts of his body. The man who breathes correctly and adequately does so as an immediate and inevitable consequence of normal and salubrious conditions of the same parts. It therefore follows that if the conditions present in the second man can be induced in the first, he will then, but not otherwise, be a correct and adequate breather. And the process by which this is achieved is simply a readjustment of the parts of the body by a new and correct use of the muscular mechanisms through the directive agent of the sphere of consciousness. This change brings about a proper mechanical advantage of all the parts concerned, and causes, thanks to the right employment of the relative machinery, such expansion and contraction of the thoracic cavity as to give atmospheric pressure its opportunity. Now here we have *(a)* the directive agent of the sphere of consciousness, and *(b)* the use of the muscular mechanisms— the combination causing certain expansions and contractions, and *the result being what is known as breathing.* It will at once be seen, therefore, that the act of breathing is not a primary, or even a secondary, part of the process, which is really *re-education of the kinaesthetic systems associated with correct bodily postures and respiration,* and will be referred to universally as such in the near future. As a matter of fact, given the perfect co-ordination of parts as required by my system, breathing is a subordinate operation which will perform itself.

I stand by every word of this to-day. Hundreds of soldiers every year have to leave the British Army on account of heart trouble directly brought about by the "drill-sergeant's chest" and its concomitant strains and rigidities. Not long ago, Mr. Punch had a picture of a young boy riding in the Row with his groom and answering that worthy's question as to how he would salute a Royal Personage—"Same as the soldiers do; hold my hand up to my hat and look as if I was going to burst"! Certainly a straw showing which way the wind blows.

These same soldiers will start on a long route march with chest "well set" and stiff. The strain of marching inevitably brings them later into an easier slouching position, which makes continuance possible, and at its worst is not so positively harmful as is the tension of the other posture.

Compare the free, loose but more healthy physical attitude of the sailor ashore with that of the "smart" soldier strutting in town like a pouter pigeon for the honour of the regiment. It is your team of sailors that is the readier and the more effective for hard work.

And but a few weeks (now years) ago I saw with dismay in a popular illustrated daily paper a truly pathetic picture of a class of schoolboys with hollowed backs and protruding chests looking like nothing so much as very ruffled pouter pigeons. And the master was commended for his zeal in producing such results by "deep breathing." (See photographs facing this page.)

Is it, I would ask, likely on the face of it that the right position in which a man or woman should stand for health's sake should be one needing positive strain to preserve? The thing is preposterous, and I am convinced that nothing can result from the application of such principles but complete chaos, physical and mental.

To return to my general theory of training, I fear I must not particularize too definitely in some directions, but my instance of right-handedness has its application. On the one hand we are willing to sacrifice reason for such a tradition and convention as this; on the other for an untried and possibly illogical idea. The defence for the latter sacrifice is generally based either on the need for enthusiasm or the necessity for proceeding by a system of trial and error. Well, as to enthusiasm, I will claim that no one is a greater enthusiast than I am myself, but I will not permit my enthusiasm to dominate my reason. One day I hope to write an account of how I arrived at the practical elucidation of my principles of conscious control, and when I do, I shall show very plainly how one of the greatest, if not *the* greatest, dangers against which I had to fight was my own enthusiasm. It is as vivid and keen to-day as it was over twenty years ago, but I should never have worked out my principles if I had allowed it to dominate my reason. Again, as to the argument pleading the necessity for empiricism, I admit also that my own methods have been, and still are, in some directions, experimental. But with regard to the "free expression" movement, I claim that the error in practice has been sufficiently demonstrated, and, further than that, I must insist that we are not justified in experimenting on children. I have never done that, inasmuch as I have realized that the error may be irreparable. Could any fault weigh heavier on a human conscience than that by which, however unwittingly, another human life had been distorted?

Wherefore, pleading on behalf of my most important client, the child of this younger generation, I demand that we shall proceed to neither of the dangerous extremes that threaten his physical and mental well-being. On the one hand we must avoid the thrusting upon him of fixed ideas, by which you may narrow his mind, for I know that when you limit him, imparting to him deliberately your own mental habits, the effects go far beyond what we are pleased to call the "formation of character." On the other hand we are not justified in leaving him entirely to himself. Whilst he has the right of choice within certain limits, he has not, unhappily, the ability to choose in his earlier years. We need not bind him to choose this or that, but we must educate him in such a way as to give him the power of choice. In Mr. Allen Upward's delightful work, *The New World,* which I have already quoted, he says: "Give the child leave to grow. Give the child leave to live. Give the child leave to hope and to hope truly.... He is the plaintiff in this case. I say that he is mankind... and his birthright is the truth." And to that I would add, " Give the child leave, also, to learn. Give him opportunity to profit by all the knowledge we can give him out of our experience. His birthright, indeed, is the truth, but we must aid him in making the discovery."

It is full time that we gave more earnest thought to this matter. I cannot in this brief outline dwell on the many phases of proper food, clothing, and physical training, and all those other points which we must consider. The kinaesthetic systems concerned with correct and healthy bodily movements and postures have become demoralized by the habits engendered in the schoolroom through the restraint enforced at a time when natural activity should have been encouraged and scientifically directed, and in the crouching positions caused by useless and irrational desk-work.

And I may note in this connection that I am continually being asked, both by friends and unknown correspondents, for my opinion concerning the correct type of chair, stool, desk, or table to be used in order to prevent the bad habits which these pieces of furniture are supposed to have caused in schools. In my replies I have tried to demonstrate that the problem is being attacked from the wrong standpoint.

Let us consider the problem in the light of common sense. Suppose, for example, that there is an ideal chair, some wonderful arrangement of perfect angles, hollows, and supports that will almost magically rectify or prevent every fault in the child's physical mechanism. Suppose further that the child finds great ease and repose when seated in this ideal chair. How, then, can he avoid suffering the tortures of all that is uncomfortable when he rides in the cars, or sits down in his own home, or visits a friend, or goes for a picnic on the river or in the woods? I see nothing else for it; when that ideal chair has been found, our child will have to carry it about with him wherever he goes.

In the second place, how is it possible for this ideal chair to be miraculously adaptable to every age and type of child? Are we to treat children as plastic lumps of clay to be fitted to the model insisted upon by the lines of our ideal chair; or are we to study and measure each individual and have a chair built to his measure, once a year, say, until he is adult?

No, what we need to do is not to educate our school furniture, but to educate our children. Give a child the ability to adapt himself within reasonable limits to his environment, and he will not suffer discomfort, nor develop bad physical habits, whatever chair or form you give him to sit upon. I say, "within reasonable limits," for it is obviously absurd to expect a Brobdingnagian child to use a Lilliputian chair. But let us waste no valuable time, thought, or invention in designing furniture, when by a smaller expenditure of those three gifts we may train the child to win its own conscious control, and rise superior to any probable limitations imposed by ordinary school fittings. For the problem to be solved in education is that same problem which needs solution in the social, political, religious, industrial, economic, ethical, aesthetic, and other spheres of progressive human activity. In every sphere of life we have for years given "effects" the significance of "causes" and have made worthy attempts to put matters right on this unsound basis.

In the case of education certain symptoms have been recognized as more or less harmful, and the whole blame has been placed upon the method or methods of education involved. For at least half a century the method of the social worker was conceived on the lines of giving money, food, and clothing to the poor, in an attempt to ameliorate their condition.

The evils of this false policy came home to them in a practical way, and nowadays the object of the social worker is to give the poor the "means whereby" of general advancement and of getting money, clothes, and food by their own efforts.

The same principle holds good in the treatment of the children. Hitherto educationalists have given them what they considered they needed. What we must do in the future is to give them the "means whereby" they may themselves satisfy their needs and command their own advancement.

The adoption of new methods is a procedure which always demands a due and proper consideration of the thing, person, or persons to which they are to be applied. Investigation along these lines would probably have revealed the real *cause* of the difficulties to be faced in the education of the child of to-day, which is that the process of civilized life has gradually changed the child's psycho-physical condition at birth. In this process much has been gained and much lost. From the educator's point of view the losses have been stupendous as compared with the gains, for the all-important kinaesthetic systems have been deteriorated by man's attempt to pass from the lower (animal) to the higher stages of the evolutionary plane while depending on a subconsciously controlled organism.

I have still very much more to say on this subject of education, and I hope to have an opportunity in the near future of elaborating my methods and of setting them out so that they may be practically and universally applied. But if by these few remarks I can arouse some interest in this world problem, I shall have done something towards its solution. It is a problem which is very urgent at the present time, and is growing more urgent every day. All that we have done up to the present time is to enforce one rule or another upon the children as an experiment, for all the rules have been rigid in their enforcement, however unscientific in their conception. In place of these rules I look for an ideal which I believe to be comparatively easy of realization. I look for, and already see, a method of training our children which shall make them masters of their own bodies; I look for a time when the child shall be so taught and trained that whatever the circumstance which shall later surround it, it will without effort be able to adapt itself to its environment, and be enabled to live its life in the enjoyment of perfect health, physical and mental. For, as I have already pointed out, man has progressed towards the higher and more complex stages of civilization. He has continued to change his habits of life and, being still far from the highest state attainable, he will continue to change. The farther he becomes removed from the primitive uncivilized stage of his evolution, the less likely is he to have the opportunity in the daily routine of his life so to exercise the physical machinery that it will be prevented from working imperfectly by the controls of instinct. "Conscious control" will enable man to adapt himself more readily to changing conditions of life. No one who looks out upon this latter-day world with discerning eyes can fail to see that the changes tend to become more rapid and more radical than ever before in the history of the world's progress. We look towards the goal, and it is best to seek the highest and be content with no less, but at the same time it is necessary that we should consider the practical detail of our journey. What follows in Parts II and III

Matthias Alexander

may seem trivial by comparison with the high endeavour I have outlined, but it is the triviality of the essential detail.

I wish to point the road still more clearly, and to show how every man and woman may learn to walk upon it.

CHAPTER VIII - EVOLUTIONARY STANDARDS AND THEIR INFLUENCE ON THE CRISIS OF 1914
15

IN the previous chapters I have dealt briefly with the fundamentals upon which our whole structure of education and civilization is based, and have attempted to point to the different tendencies developed by the individual in the struggle to progress upon this basis. At the same time I have indicated that which I am confident is the only true fundamental upon which mankind in a state of civilization may progress and evolve to a condition commanding freedom for all time from those limiting, narrowing, and debasing qualities which belong to the animal spheres of existence.

It seems to me that the present world crisis indicates that this is the psychological moment to make a wide application of my principles, though my reader may consider that I should not enter the debatable ground of hypothesis in a work which has been devoted, up to this point, to arguments almost entirely drawn from personal experiences and observation.

I have dealt with the fundamentals employed in the development of the child and the adult, and I have postulated that the evolutionary progress from childhood to adolescence, and on through the vicissitudes of life which follow, is determined by the process adopted, the ratio of progress being in accordance with the standard of efficacy of this process, and that this principle of evolution applies equally to a nation.

It then devolves upon us to consider the different processes adopted by different nations, in order to gauge accurately their different stages of evolution and their possibilities of growth and development towards real individual and national progress.

After centuries of endeavour in the direction of progress in accordance with well-defined processes, founded upon approved educational, religious, economic, political, industrial, ethical, and aesthetic principles, and after a century of unprecedented progress in

---

[15] This chapter was written at the end of the 1914-1918 war, but the analysis made in it is still fundamentally valid for the crisis of our present time.

the realm of Arts and Sciences, we are faced with the spectacle, in a supposedly civilized nation, of a debauched kinaesthesia which has manifested itself in such a display of savage instincts as will present us in the eyes of a more highly evolved universe as plunged in the depths of barbarism.[16]

During the past three years the people of the world have been shocked and stirred by events which even four years ago were considered impossible in the stage of civilization then reached. In consequence, we find that a special and earnest endeavour is being made to solve problems of vital importance which have a bearing upon the future development and cultivation of the potentialities of mankind.

It is therefore essential to recognize that we have reached a point in the process called civilization which will be recorded as one of the most critical and vital in the world's history.

At this moment the great nations of Europe are emerging from the most terrific conflict of force ever recorded.

The happenings of these years of war must influence our present and future opinion of the value of our educational, political, moral, social, industrial, religious, and other principles where the progress of man is concerned, as he passes from the animal plane of his evolution to those higher planes for which he is undoubtedly destined.

The conclusions thus reached will so influence the future welfare of mankind that the facts from which these conclusions are deduced demand the most serious attention and study of every human being.

It is therefore essential that we make an earnest endeavour to discover fundamentals. In this connection we must consider the available evidence concerning the cause or causes of this conflict in Europe which has shaken our boasted advancement in civilization to its very roots. What does this recrudescence of barbarity mean when

---

[16] As I re-read this in 1945, the papers are full of the indescribable brutalities of the German concentration camps.—F. M. A. against the more highly evolved races, the struggle of an openminded, mobile idealism for the supremacy of the individual against a narrow-minded, rigid, material automatism which entails the suppression of the individual and the obliteration of his reason in the supposed interests of the State.

viewed with an open and unprejudiced mind in its relation to the future of those principles which alone make for the real mental, physical, and spiritual growth of mankind in progressive civilization?

It signifies a tremendous clash of opposing forces, a desperate conflict between the lowly evolved peoples of the world as

Let us take, then, a general comparative view of the compelling psycho-physical forces in the life of primitive and civilized nations up to the crisis.

In Primitive Nations. The compelling forces were chiefly physical and subconscious. The very essentials of life depended almost entirely on brute force. Daily experiences gave a keen edge to savage instincts and unbridled passions, to an automatic development which opposed the cultivation of the faculty of adaptability to new environments. Even the spheres of courage were limited, and when confronted with the unusual these peoples quaked like cowards, and fled panic-stricken from the unaccustomed, as in the case of the negroes in the Southern States of America when the men of the Ku-Klux Klan pursued them on horseback dressed in white.

In Civilized Nations. The compelling forces have become less and less physical and less subconscious than in the case of primitive nations, but the advance from the physical to the mental and from the subconscious to the conscious has not been adequate or sufficiently comprehensive to establish the mental and conscious principles as the chief compelling forces in the progress of the nation or even of the individual. The essentials of life do not depend on brute force, and daily experiences become less and less associated with factors which make for the development of savage instincts and unbridled passion, or automatic development. But experience has proved that civilized nations have failed to come through the ordeal of adaptation to the ever-changing environment of civilization with satisfactory results. The spheres of courage are still more or less limited, and when brought suddenly face to face with the unusual and unexpected, people still exhibit a tendency to panic and loss of control. The progress made by civilized nations from the primitive state to the present has not been upon comprehensive lines. The result has been that the majority of the activities of the nation have been limited, and in those few activities where the widening influence held sway, the freedom became licence and led to over-compensation. This condition was sufficiently harmful as long as it applied to the individual and to individual effort, the individual being more or less held in check by collective opinion; but when it applied to the nation and to national effort, that nation which ignored the opinion of other nations developed unchecked, and the national decision to stifle the individual, body and soul, if it seemed to be for the welfare of the State, constituted the most powerful force in the prevention of progress on the evolutionary plane.

For this decision, once it became the result of national conception, carried with it the most damaging and impossible of all mental processes in the sphere of true evolutionary advancement. In the first place the national decision was the result of an erroneous national conception, the outcome of what I have called, for the want of a better name, "manufactured premises."

Manufactured premises are the forerunners of unsound and delusive deductions—a stultification of reason—and demand the cultivation of a form of self-hypnotism which is fatal to national or individual progress.

A few observant people noted this dangerous habit even in the early literature of the German nation, and watched with keen interest its cultivation in all spheres of activity in recent years. This explains the stupendous failure of German judgment in all matters of national and international importance, of the impossibility of the peoples of that nation to see anything from any other point of view but their own, of their crass stupidity in gauging the psychology of other nations, and particularly that of the British nation.

In the foregoing we have fundamentals worthy of consideration. They must occupy the attention of all thinking people who wish to make a contribution towards the uplifting of mankind and the establishment of a standard of reasoned guidance and control which should make another barbarous conflict unthinkable and therefore impossible.

Naturally, every nation is ready enough with a more or less humane reason for its madness. Self-protection, an altruistic regard for the rights of smaller nations, a sense of high duty towards mankind at large—all these pleas have been urged as explaining the single principle which has drawn this or that nation into the whirlpool. And each and every nation must surely have pleaded liberty as their excuse at some time or another, liberty being one of those adaptable terms that may be used to mean almost anything. Before the war Germany was maintaining a right for "liberty" of expansion, a defensive use of the word that has hardly anything in common with its use at the present time.

On the other hand, philosophers, economists, psychologists, commercial experts, and the public at large have been busy with a dozen other theories of the primary causes of the war. We have heard much talk of race hatred, of business rivalry, of high commercial and political intrigues, and a dozen other influences, and all of them have been put forward at one time or another as the sole reason for the present welter of blood and fury. We have, in fine, so many reasons from which to choose that we may be quite sure no single one of them can possibly afford us an inclusive and adequate explanation.

But I will go still farther than that. For I maintain on grounds which I find logically unshakeable, that if we admit, as seems the only sensible course, that something of all these reasons and excuses has entered into the conditions producing such awful results, we must still seek some explanation of the preceding state that made these conditions possible. All our reasons, in fact, are mere effects, and we are groping for our primary cause among resultant phenomena. We can never solve our problem by such a method as this. We might as well hope to find the origin of a child by dissecting its limbs and intestines. Our only hope is to shift our viewpoint, to cease our muddled examination of the details just in front of us, and try to see our problem in the broad terms of one who can stand back and see life moving through the centuries.

With all people, in all spheres of life, we know only too well that certain mental and physical manifestations give an absolute clue to their character, to their aims in life, their ideals, and, what is more to the point, to the stage they have reached in the process called evolution.

Incidentally, I would point out that education as generally understood, even when it implies the most up-to-date methods, does not necessarily mean progress on the evolutionary plane, any more than ability as a linguist need denote a high standard of mentality.

This applies also to most arts, and particularly to those where music and dancing are concerned. The lower the stage of evolution, within certain limits, the greater the appeal of music and dancing.

When we review the history and general progress of humanity we find the instincts and traits of the animal—the bruteforce principle— predominating at certain stages. If we go back far enough we find that there was a stage when it was always predominant.

Therefore, a test as to the ratio of progress of nations on the evolutionary plane is to be found in their tendency and desire to advance beyond that stage where the mental and physical forces, which should only belong as inherited instincts to the brute animals and savages, hold sway; and with this in view, if we take a survey of the history, ideals, habits of life, mental outlook, and general tendencies of the German nation, it will show conclusively that these self-hypnotized people approximated too closely to the lower animals and savages in their mode and chief aims of life.

The great and noble ideals and aims of mankind making for progress towards the more highly evolved states were cast aside for the unreasoning, brutal, and ignoble principles which make for the debasement of man's elevating potentialities, and hold him a slave to the cruel and lowly evolved state of the primitive creatures. That any nation or nations should deliberately adopt, as their highest ideals and aims, brute force in all its hideous aspects, desecration of mind, body, and soul for the State, justification of criminal instincts and acts if employed on behalf of the State, destruction, rape and plunder, murder and torture to terrify innocent civilians; that they should adopt, in short, the brutal principle that "Might is Right" in that special national form in which it has been manifested in the last half century and directed towards what is now known as "Militarism"— all this is surely proof positive that they have progressed but little on the upward evolutionary stage from the state occupied by the brute beast and the savage. The criminal aspect of the outrage of all that right-thinking human beings hold dear is intensified by the fact that the nations which perpetrated the deed were among the most prosperous of the world, and enjoyed, as aliens, the same privileges as the subjects of those nations whose hospitality and confidence they abused.

The nations bearing the brunt of the struggle against this outburst of primitive brutal instincts and desires have long since reached a stage in their evolution which made the methods of Attila unthinkable. If forced into war, they conducted it on the evolved plane of the human, and not that of the animal. They treated their captives as honourable men and extended to them every conceivable consideration within their power. Prior to this war the ideals and aims of these nations were the antithesis of those of their lowly-evolved enemies, and they were ideals and aims which made for the right to live in peace with all other nations. They aimed at the reduction of armaments, and gave practical proof of their aims. They opened their ports and their markets to their present enemies and gave them a free hand in every respect in all spheres of activity. They had no desire to beat down the ideals and principles which make for the ennoblement of mankind, they had no wish to dominate the world by brute force and to establish a system of living and a form of conduct which grind the individual into a mere heartless unreasoning automaton, rigid-brained, driven like an animal, and not daring to claim even his soul as his own.

For many years prior to the crisis of 1914 we listened to the blatant outbursts of German professors and other educated authorities of that nation concerning its superiority to other nations. We were asked to believe that certain individuals of that nationality had reached the stage of the superman. These unfortunate and deluded people have for some time been cursed with this obsession.

Thinking men and women of other nations listened and wondered when these claims were made concerning the supermen, and after examining the evidence advanced to support these claims became convinced that they were not justified. The stupendous failure of the supposed supermen in every sphere of mental and physical activity in the present war proves the correctness of these convictions.

It seems inconceivable that supermen could so have guided and directed the whole national energy of Germany that it became more and more narrowed—like the German mind— until it concentrated almost solely upon the stupid conception of the domination of the world by Germany. To this end, the national energy was diverted chiefly into two channels: COMMERCIAL INDUSTRY AND MILITARISM

One of the great features connected with the former was the extraordinary development of machinery, which demanded for its

Matthias Alexander

successful pursuance that the individual should be subjected to the most harmful systems of automatic training.

The standardized parts of the machine made demands which tended to stereotype the human machine. The limitations of human activity, mental and physical, reached the maximum. The power to continue work under such conditions depended on a process of deterioration in the individual. He was slowly but surely being robbed of the possibility of development. The very soul of man was crushed to foster an industrial process which was to provide the sinews of the war machine, to support that curse called militarism, and the demoralization of Germany came chiefly through that nation's conceptions of militarism, which, in the first and last analysis, stands for the worst manifestation of those savage instincts and unbridled passions associated with the lowest stages of primitive race development.

The horrible results of the sum total of the national madness which the foregoing represents are now revealed before us, for to Germany this militarism constituted a rigid plan, a system, and a world-philosophy.

She is convinced, against all the evidence, that her plan, system, or philosophy, is so undeniably right as to constitute an absolute. As a nation she has no mobility, no poise. She is influenced by a stultifying idea, the perfection of her own "Kultur" (a word more properly translated as a civilization than by the word "culture" as used in the English or American sense). She is, in fact, just as badly co-ordinated, as unable to follow the true mandate of reason, as any individual who is dominated by a fixed idea.

For the trouble is that when reason is so far held in check that it loses its power of denial, it must have lost its power of control. The original "idea" formulated in the conscious mind has sunk so deep into the subconscious that it cannot be changed except under the influence of some stronger outside power. For nearly fifty years Germany, in her schools, her gymnasiums, her universities, her civic and her political life, has been inculcating a rigid and mentally demoralizing system, and she is suffering now—as the monomaniac in private life must suffer—for her particular form of insanity.

Even in the conduct of her great campaign, this weakness of hers has begun to defeat her. She has lost the power of adaptability in military matters. She repeats the faults of her original plan, despite the endless illustrations that have been afforded by her Western antagonists that that plan can be very considerably bettered. No doubt the Higher Command may realize in some instances the weakness of the old method in conditions that have been immensely modified since August 1914, but they are impotent to change, in a year or in a decade, the effect of their own teaching on the millions of Germany's army. The massed attack, for example, has been demonstrated to be a disastrous failure—a single well-placed machine-gun can defeat it—but Germany's soldiers will not advance in a scattered attack. They have learnt to depend on the nearness of their comrades. Separate a German battalion and it has neither confidence nor courage.

Returning now to my single reason for the cause of the present war, I feel that the explanation has already been given. Granted a nation educated and trained as Germany has been, some explosion was inevitable sooner or later. If we have in our midst an individual suffering from a fixed idea, he must in time become intolerable to us. Never in the history of the world have thought and the tendency to organization been more fluid than they were in the first years of the twentieth century. Yet one great and powerful nation interfered with us at every turn, impeding the flow of liberal thought by her obsession with the ideas of her own greatness and the omnipotence of her military machine. Nevertheless the other nations of Europe adapted themselves within limits to the demands of this rigid mechanism in their midst. And it may be that these very powers of endurance and adaptability hastened the crisis. They were regarded by the monomaniacs of Germany as signs of weakness, and just as their own philosopher Nietzsche went mad by concentration on his own invariable theme, so at last Germany crossed the bounds of sanity, imbued with a crazy belief in her own omnipotence. She ran amuck in the wide streets of Europe, and even yet she has not realized her own madness. I seriously question whether she will come to anything like a proper realization of that madness in the present generation. She has allowed a habit of mind to become fixed; and it has fallen into the realms of her subconsciousness. We must treat her as mad, but she is nevertheless to be pitied.

Matthias Alexander

POSTSCRIPT

It has been suggested to me that the subject-matter of this chapter, as specially written in 1918 for the enlarged edition of this book, "dates" too much to be applicable to events and conditions at the present time. I am well aware of the changes in general outlook that world-wide happenings have forced upon us in many spheres of life since the chapter was written; nevertheless, with the exception of certain small omissions and alterations which are being made in the text in recognition of this changed outlook, it is being reprinted in its original form for the following reasons:

Recent events have shown that I was amply justified in the predictions I made in this chapter—viz., that the nature of the human element in Germany, and the attitude towards it of the human element in other nations, was such that it would lead inevitably to a further crisis, and I wish here to reassert my conviction that unless means are adopted for bringing about a basic change in the reactions of the individual human being in every country, a repetition of the present tragic frustration of human endeavour must be expected.

The same self-imposed slavery of habit, which dominated the thought and actions of mankind, both individually and nationally, between the years 1914-1918, still dominates human reaction, as manifested in the years just passed, 1939-1945. This form of slavery has been revealed especially in the persistence of certain harmful trends, leading to fixation, both national and international, mass hysteria, and, most significant of all, perhaps, in this connexion, in direction and judgment which has been so faulty and ill-advised in the matter of relative values concerning human relations and man's activities in general, that it has frustrated his best-intentioned efforts in almost every field of activity.

As the arguments, conclusions, and predictions stated in the following extracts have been justified by world-wide happenings, I think the reader may find them interesting: *The British Medical Journal,* June 18, 1932. Extract from letter to the Editor from Dr. Peter Macdonald, of York.

> "Man's control over things—steam and explosives, and atoms and space—has outrun his power over himself to use that command wisely. No proof of this is needed beyond the tragic

conditions of the world today, and it is because Alexander will in time be recognized as the pioneer worker in establishing the conscious control of the use of the self that he will be given his place in history as the seer he is, on the condition, a quite uncertain one, that civilization lasts so long."

The Medical Press and Circular, July 18-, 1945. Extract from article entitled "Knowing How to Stop," by Dr. Wilfred Barlow.

"In teaching the individual to maintain harmony and stability in the face of all the stimulation of the modern world, Alexander seeks to bring into play the one faculty which marks us off from the rest of organic life, the ability to *stop* and *choose:* he seeks to reinstate this one weapon of self-defence, the ability to say *no.* It is the loss of this ability to say *no* which is responsible for the instability and disharmony which characterises modern man both in war and peace: for the war is only an accentuation of the raucous stimulating peace-time world—a world which flashes us a hundred different commands and directions in a single day, conflicting directions which make it essential for us to discriminate and to choose."

Extract from *Constructive Conscious Control of the Individual,* Part I.

"I venture to predict that before we can unravel the horribly tangled skein of our present existence, we must come to a full STOP, and return to conscious, simple living, believing in the unity underlying all things, and acting in a practical way in accordance with the laws and principles involved.

In the midst of a world-wide tragedy such as we are witnessing at the present time, a tragedy which seems to have been increasing instead of decreasing in its intensity since the declaration of the Armistice and the work of the peace-makers, surely it behoves every individual to stop— and I mean this in its fullest sense—and reconsider every particle of supposed knowledge, particularly ' psychological ' knowledge, derived from his general education, from his religious, political, moral, ethical, social, legal and economic training, and ask himself the plain, straightforward question, 'Why do I believe these things?' 'By what process of reasoning did I arrive at these conclusions?'"

END OF PART I

PART II - CONSCIOUS GUIDANCE AND CONTROL

EDUCATION
"It is because the body is a machine that education is possible. Education is the formation of habits, a superinducing of an artificial organization upon the natural organization of the body; so that acts, which at first require a conscious effort, eventually become unconscious and mechanical."—HUXLEY.

RE-EDUCATION
"It is because the body is a machine that (RE)-education is possible. (RE)-education is the formation of (NEW AND CORRECT) habits, a (Re-INSTATING OF THE CORRECT) artificial organization upon the natural organization of the body; so that acts, which at first require conscious effort, eventually become unconscious and mechanical."

INTRODUCTION TO PART II
IN the first part of this volume I have endeavoured to explain the general principle which underlies my work. I will now present my proposition from a slightly different angle, as it were, to ensure a clearer view of it—that is, I shall deal with it in the light of its practical application to the acts of everyday life.

I trust I may do something to convince thinking men and women that conscious control is essential to man's satisfactory progress in civilization, and that the properly directed use of such control will enable the individual to stand, sit, walk, breathe, digest, and in fact live with the least possible expenditure of vital energy. This will ensure the highest standard of resistance to disease. When this desirable stage of our evolution is reached the cry of physical deterioration may no longer be heard.

I will write out as concisely, as definitely, and as boldly as possible, my claims and my main argument. In a second part I have added some more discursive notes and comments which I trust will meet the many requests I have received for further light on certain points in my former book.

My experience of the past fifty-one years enables me to set down

Matthias Alexander

my convictions in terms that do not admit of any doubt or
uncertainty. My conclusions on the urgent question of physical
decadence have not been formulated in haste. They are deductions
from a long series of striking results and observed facts, and, frankly, I
consider them so important that I cannot hesitate to deliver my
message in a tone which may appear to some to savour of over-
confidence. So be it!

CHAPTER I - SYNOPSIS OF CLAIM

1. MY first claim is that psycho-physical guidance by conscious control, when applied as a universal principle to "living," constitutes an unfailing preventive for diseases mental or physical, malformations, and loss of general efficiency. It is commonly considered that these conditions are brought about by such evils of civilization as the limitation of energy, and by that loss of so-called "natural conditions" which civilization entails.

It is my earnest belief that the intelligent recognition of the principles essential to guidance by conscious control are essential to the full mental and physical development of the human race. Due consideration will convince even the sceptical that if mankind is to evolve to the higher stages of mental and physical perfection, he must be guided by these principles. They alone will bring men and women of to-day to the highest state of wellbeing, enabling them to grapple effectively with the problems of the day in the world of thought and action, gradually widening the dividing line which separates civilized mankind from the animal kingdom.

There is no sphere of human activity, of human feeling or philosophy where the adoption of the principles of conscious guidance and control would not bring invaluable benefits.

At present man is held in bondage by many subconscious instincts which enslave the animal kingdom, the savage, and the semi-savage. Let me illustrate this. Animals and savages become immediately unbalanced when they experience the unusual, as for instance when they see an express train dash along for the first time. Such a new experience would cause the bravest animal to become overwhelmed with that degree of fear which momentarily suspends his normal guidance by instinct. So also with the savage, who would be equally unbalanced by an experience of this kind. In most spheres of normal life, he, like the animal, depends on instinctive guiding principles which act with perfect balance in accustomed circumstances. In the face of the unusual, however, he is unable to meet suddenly the requirements of a new environment. To meet these he needs reasoned, conscious guidance which is the outcome of the habit of conscious control, and marks the dividing line between the animal kingdom, where instinct is the guide, and the human kingdom, where its members are in communication with reason.

The mental and physical Mutations and imperfections of men and women of the present day make it impossible for them to meet satisfactorily the great majority of the. requirements of their present environment, and render them quite incapable of making the best of their capabilities in any new environment. These instinctive guiding principles, not even perfectly balanced, as in the case of the savage and the animal, are miserably insufficient to meet the conditions of the modern world with its ever-changing environment. Yet it is upon these instincts that men and women rely, to the detriment of their mental and physical attainments.

2. My next claim is that the limitations and imperfections referred to above, as well as cancer, appendicitis, bronchitis, tuberculosis, etc., are too often permitted to remain uneradicated and frequently undetected, and so to develop in consequence of the failure to recognize that the real cause of the development of such diseases is to be found in the erroneous preconceived ideas of the persons immediately concerned, ideas which affect the organism in the manner described in Part I of this book.

The Only experience which the average man or woman has in the use of the different parts of the human organism is through his or her subconsciousness. The result is a subconscious direction which in the imperfectly co-ordinated person is based on bad experiences and on the erroneous preconceived ideas before mentioned. Small wonder, then, that such direction is faulty and leads to the development of serious defects and imperfections. With this erroneous direction even the attempt to carry out a simple action in accordance with subconscious habit is fraught with danger, for it invariably affects in a detrimental manner other parts of the subject's organism which have nothing to do with the particular act Or acts attempted. For instance, in the subconsciously controlled person the attempt to lengthen the neck is invariably preceded by a movement of the eyes in an upward or downward direction. Wrong use of the eyes in this or some similar manner too frequently is the forerunner of what eventually develops into an established habit, often causing an unnecessary and undue strain of the eyes which seriously impairs their efficiency, and which in the ordinary way of life leads to the specific treatment of these organs. It is obvious, however, that what is needed in such a case is the eradication of the erroneous preconceived idea and harmful habits, thereby removing gradually the undue and unnecessary strain upon the organs of sight. This will enable them to regain their lost efficiency and it is almost certain that specific treatment of any kind on orthodox lines will be unnecessary. In consequence of faulty guidance misdirected energies are not confined to one part of the organism. They affect the hands, arms, shoulders, legs, thorax, hips, knees, ankles, and other parts of the organism, frequently causing strain and interference with the functioning of the different organs, and finally seriously injuring them. To support this second claim I bring forward the following arguments:

(a) Till now little or no attention on a practical psychophysical basis has been given to the vital and harmful influence of this faulty direction (of subconscious origin) and of the erroneous preconceived ideas and faulty posture associated therewith. Under such influences the subject can hardly fail to cultivate a wrong mental attitude towards life in general and towards the art of living (evolving satisfactorily), especially in regard to the primary causation of the defects which may be present or which may develop eventually, but also in regard to the essential laws connected with the eradication of these defects.

(b) Owing to the lack of distinction between reasoned (conscious) and unreasoned (subconscious or partly conscious) actions, the subject suffers from various forms of mental and physical delusions, notably with regard to the physical acts he performs. Incidentally it should be pointed out that if this is true of the ordinary acts of everyday life, how much more so of those physical acts which may be necessary to meet the demands of some new environment! As a striking instance of delusion in physical acts let us take the case of a man who believes himself to be merely overcoming what he regards as essential inertia, when he is really fighting the resistance of undue antagonistic muscular action exerted by himself, a resistance of which he is not consciously aware. In all such cases there is a constant conflict between two great forces, the one (subconscious) destined to exercise supreme directive powers during the early stages of human evolution, the other (conscious) to supersede this limited direction and finally to prove the reliable guide through the higher and highest stages of the great evolutionary scheme which leads to the full enjoyment of his potentialities. It must be remembered that the former became firmly established during centuries of subconscious direction, holding undisputed sway until the first glimmering of reasoned conscious guidance came in its crudest form to disturb its power, a power which it is destined one day to overthrow. In the present stage of our mental and physical progress the conflict continues with gradually increasing energy, and while the conflict is being waged the subject is influenced first in one direction by the dictates of his subconsciousness (called by some "instinct," by others "intuition"), and then in another by his awakened conscious powers which he is gradually but slowly developing. Of the real significance of this conflict he has, unfortunately, no true realization. At the same time he undoubtedly feels the force of these two influences as conflicting energies, but only in a dim, mysterious way. He is swayed first by one force and then by the other, as happens when we hear a man or woman say, "Well, that seems the thing to do, but I feel that I shouldn't do it."

Very often he does what he feels instead of what seems to be the correct thing, and, moreover, the former is very frequently right. This is not surprising, seeing that the subconscious instinct in us is much more developed than the conscious faculty. But granting the subconscious its fullest degree of merit, we are forced to recognize its serious limitations in the mode of life (civilization) with its ever-changing environment which human progress demands. We must have a guiding principle without these limitations, to enable us to adapt ourselves much more quickly to the new environments which are inevitable in the progress of civilization towards its legitimate goal.

We must have something more reasoned and definite than that which subconscious direction offers, and so we come to the need of reasoned guidance. Up to the present neither of these forms of direction really reaches the mind as a definite tangible idea consciously conceived. This is because of the fundamental principles upon which subconscious direction has been built up, and in consequence of the undeveloped condition of conscious guidance. Furthermore, the subject has not yet made any serious attempt to analyse these two forces, of whose particular workings he is but dimly aware. The fundamental principle which we call evolution demands that every human being shall be enabled to make this analysis, so that he may differentiate between the impulses springing from his subconsciousness (instinct-inhibition) and the conceptions created in his reasoning conscious mind.

The subject will thus cultivate the habit of distinguishing between reasoned and unreasoned actions, and this will at once tend to the prevention of mental and physical delusions in all directions, notably in regard to his physical acts in old or new environments.

(c) Whilst these delusions remain, the subject will continue to perform wrong or detrimental actions, for as long as his settled mental attitude towards such actions remains unchanged he will believe that he is performing them in a correct manner. It is owing to this involuntary, and on his part unrecognized, misapprehension, that many malformations and inefficiencies become established, which sooner or later may lead to definite disease. The popular misconception of the subject's responsibility in the matter leads him to be commonly pitied as for unavoidable defects, whereas it is of the first importance that he should realize the responsibility is his, and his alone. He must be made aware that such defects arise from his own fault and are the outcome of his ignorance or wilful neglect.

Once this new mental attitude is firmly established there is hope for the afflicted person, and he will have the satisfaction of knowing that he is, as it were, working out his own salvation on common-sense practical lines, devoid of pernicious sympathy, face to face with real facts, and stimulated by a principle which cannot fail to secure the very best efforts in the right direction of which any ordinary person is capable.

(d) It is essential, in the necessary re-education of the subject through conscious guidance and control, that in every case the "means whereby" rather than the "end" should be held in mind. As long as the "end" is held in mind instead of the "means," the muscular act, or series of acts, will always be performed in accordance with the mode established by old habits. When each stage of the series essential to the "means whereby" is correctly apprehended by the conscious mind of the subject, the old habits can be broken up, and every muscular action can be consciously directed until the new and correct guiding sensations have established the new proper habits, which in their turn become subconscious, but on a more highly evolved plane.

In effect these new habits ensure conditions which give new life to, and maintain in a high state of efficiency, every organ of the body, the automatic functions being reacted upon by the consciously controlled energies. By my system of obtaining the position of *"mechanical advantage,"* [17] a perfect system of natural internal massage is rendered possible, such as never before has been attained by orthodox methods, a system which is extraordinarily beneficial in breaking up toxic accumulation; thus avoiding evils which arise from auto-intoxication.

The position of mechanical advantage, which may or may not be a normal position, is the position which gives the teacher the opportunity to bring about quickly with his own hands a co-ordinated condition in the subject. Such co-ordination gives to the pupil an experience of the proper use of a part or parts, in the imperfect use of which may be found the primary cause of the defects present. It is by the repetition of such experiences of the proper use of his organism that the pupil is enabled to reproduce the sensation and to employ the same in what would ordinarily be considered an abnormal position (of mechanical advantage) affords the teacher an opportunity to establish the mental and physical guiding principles which enable

---

[17] A simple, practical example of what is meant by obtaining the position of mechanical advantage may be given. Let the subject sit as far back in a chair as possible. The teacher, having decided upon the orders necessary for the elongation of the spine, the freedom of the neck (i.e., requisite natural laxness), and other conditions desirable for the particular case in hand, will then ask the pupil to rehearse those orders mentally, at the same time that he himself renders assistance by the skilful use of his hands. Then, holding with one hand one or two books against the inner back of the chair, he will rely upon the pupil mentally rehearsing the orders necessary to maintain and improve the conditions present, while he, with the other hand placed upon the pupil's shoulder, causes the body gradually to incline backwards until its weight is taken by the back of the chair. The shoulder-blades will, of course, be resting against the books. The position thus secured is one of a number which I employ and which for want of a better name I refer to as a position of "mechanical advantage."

the pupil after a short time to repeat the co-ordination with the same perfection in a normal position.

I maintain in this connection that any case of incipient appendicitis may be treated successfully by these methods. Further, when this position of mechanical advantage has been attained through the employment of the first principles of conscious guidance and control, a rigid thorax may regain mobility, no matter what the age of the subject, and full thoracic expansion and contraction may be acquired and, with the minimum of effort, maintained. During the practical process by which the thoracic elasticity and maximum intrathoracic capacity are gradually established, the body of the subject is at the same time readjusted, and mental principles are inculcated which will enable him to maintain the improved conditions in posture and co-ordination which are being set up, and which will secure the normal and necessary abdominal pressure in the right direction, thus constituting a natural form of massage of the digestive organs which is maintained during the ordinary actions of everyday life.

3.   I am able to re-adjust and to teach others to re-adjust the human machine with the hands; to mould the body, as it were, into its proper shape, and with an open-minded pupil it is possible to remove many defects in a few minutes, as, for example, to change entirely the production of a voice, its quality and power.

4.   In prescribing the principles of conscious guidance and control, we are dealing not with an epidemic of physical or mental degeneracy, but with a stage in the progress of the human race from the subconscious and instinctive to the conscious and reasoned command of the whole human mechanism. In other words, we have reached a stage in the process of civilization where demands are being made which we are unable to meet satisfactorily, and with the serious results which may be seen on every hand, results from which we can escape only by passing from those primitive modes of guidance which approximate too closely to those of the animal kingdom where the greater potentialities of the human being remain latent. The suggested adoption of conscious guidance and control as a universal principle on the lines heretofore outlined will enable us to move slowly but with gradually increasing speed towards those higher psycho-physical spheres which will separate the animal and human kingdoms by a deep gulf, and mankind will then enjoy the blessings which will be the natural result of capacities fully

Matthias Alexander

developed.

CHAPTER II - THE ARGUMENT

THE marked tendency towards physical degeneracy among the men and women of all civilized races has been the constant theme of physiologists, therapeutists, and other specialists; endless explanations have been put forward to account for it, and countless remedies suggested to counteract it. In this question, as in the details of medicine and surgery, the general inclination of the human mind is always towards a treatment of epidemic symptoms, towards vague generalizations in the diagnosis and treatment of individual symptoms, whether the word "individual" in this case refers to a specific sufferer or a correlated class of diseases, towards a regard of effects rather than of causes.

As a reaction against this long-accepted method of dealing with individual symptoms by differentiated treatment, there has arisen a great diversity of so-called "mind-healers," whose *a priori* methods and lack of any clearly conceived system have brought their efforts into disrepute. Such were the conditions which over twenty years ago I sought to understand, believing—as I still do—that the whole human race was at some great psycho-physical turning-point in its history, and that if the true nature of this evolutionary stage could be understood, it might and should be possible to direct man's physical and mental progression, and so combat, and in time eliminate, a thousand evils which seem to have no counterpart in the world of the lower animals, save in very exceptional cases.

In embarking upon this inquiry I realized from the outset that I was dealing not with a world-wide epidemic, but with a stage of progress, and that it was essential therefore that I should at once discard all theories which advocated, implicitly or explicitly, a return to similar conditions. Evolution knows no such return to extinction. The species must go forward to triumphant perfection, or give place to a more dominant, more complete, self-controlled type.

Now if man as an animal, with an animal body differing little in anatomical structure from other families of the order of 117 Primates, is yet differentiated physically by a susceptibility to disease and bodily degeneration, which, save in very exceptional cases, finds little or no parallel in the lower animals, we must determine the prime cause of such differentiation. The solution of

Matthias Alexander

the problem which is commonly put forward, and which has found
support in the body calling themselves in England and in the United
States "Eugenists," I cannot accept as universal. This theory rests
mainly on the contention that in the human polity the physical
struggle for existence has ceased to have effect, that the unfit are
permitted to produce offspring equally with the fit, and that for the
natural selection imposed by circumstances which are fatal to the weak
we must substitute an arbitrary selection in order to maintain the
high efficiency of the natural type. Though I am in sympathy with
many principles of Eugenics, I reject this theory as a universal one.
It is inconsistent with the great and inspiring ideal of the progress of
the human race towards a mental and bodily perfection. If we believe
in the idea of a Purpose running through life, unfolding itself to each
successive generation and expressing itself in the terms of human
experience; if, in other words, we believe in any scientific theory of
development, in any large scheme of progress, it is impossible to accept
a theory which assumes the lack of adaptability in man's physical
body to thrive in the conditions which have grown up around him, or
to enter its true and natural kingdom of perfect soundness. If we
postulate that a third of civilized humanity is unfit to continue the
race, we can only conclude that man's physical evolution has proved
a failure, and that the race is doomed ultimately to extinction. And,
in the last analysis, it is inconceivable that the prime instinct and
desire for reproduction can be overruled at the dictates of any small
body of men, or even that such a method, if possible, could be
productive of any highly desirable results.

Wherefore I take my stand firmly on the ground that the body
of civilized man is capable not only of continuing the struggle for
existence but of rising to a higher potentiality. So, returning to the
point of differentiation between man and the lower animals, I am
now convinced that we must seek for the cause of this physical
degeneration not in the pressure of new circumstances of life, but in
the progress from one state of being to the next. I maintain that in
order to discover the solution of this twofold problem of universal
disease and its universal remedy, we must look to this enormous
growth of reasoning power, and to the consciousness and realization
of the means whereby the desired effect can be obtained. For the
animal and the lower races of mankind do not perform physical acts

118

by any process of reason. They are the servants of that strange directing law which governs the flower in its curiously ingenious devices to ensure cross-fertilization, no less than the higher mammalia in the rules of their gregarious societies, the law for which we have found no better term than Instinct. It is this "instinct" which guides all the nervous muscular mechanisms of the animal's anatomical structure, and is traceable as the motive in all functional processes. But in the physical economy of mankind this instinct is actually at war with, and is ever being controlled and superseded by conscious, directive reason.

The number of man's instinctive actions grows ever more limited, (1) as the result of a complete change of habit, and (2) more noticeably, as the outcome of a mental evolution which prompts him continually to seek a cause for every action, to analyse and endeavour to comprehend the secret springs of his being. Moreover, civilization, with its multitudinous problems of life and its perpetual interplay of personalities, demands even in the minutiae of physical action a constant reasoning, a deliberate and comparatively rapid adaptation to surroundings such as instinct is quite unable to provide. Thus man's whole body is a polity ruled by two governors whose dictates are not invariably consistent one with the other; and one governor is frequently disobeyed at the expense of the other. This fact, indeed, is obvious when it is thus considered, but we have to determine the possible outcome. There are three alternatives. The first, a return to the sole guidance of instinct, is unthinkable. The second, the continuance of this dual government, is the very condition which has led to the evils we seek to remedy. There remains the third—namely, that man's physical evolution points to progress along the road of reasoned, conscious guidance and control. It was this last conclusion which over twenty years ago led me to investigate and to practise the means by which this conscious guidance and control could be obtained, so as to apply it to the eradication and prevention of human ills, and to the maintenance of the body in a high degree of physical perfection.

CHAPTER III - THE PROCESSES OF CONSCIOUS GUIDANCE AND CONTROL

THE formulation of the method of conscious guidance and control arises in practice from a close study of the imperfect uses of the mental and physical mechanisms of the human organism. Since, as has been shown, conscious guidance and control is necessary and is being practised to some extent, inefficiently, by every civilized man and woman, it is essential that its principle should be thoroughly understood. The method is based firstly on the understanding of the co-ordinated uses of the muscular mechanisms, and secondly, on the complete acceptance of the hypothesis that each and every movement can be consciously directed and controlled.

In re-educating the individual, therefore, the first effort must be directed to the education of the conscious mind. The words "re-educating" and "re-education" have a specific meaning. In the individual the normal processes of education in the use of the anatomical structure are conducted subconsciously, certain instincts commanding certain functions, whilst other functions are conducted deliberately. The effects of this haphazard process have either to be elaborated or broken down, according to the defects established by misuse of the mechanisms, and the first step in re-education is that of establishing in the pupil's mind the connection which exists between cause and effect in every function of the human body.

In the performance of any muscular action by conscious guidance and control there are four essential stages:

(1) The conception of the movement required;

(2) The inhibition of erroneous preconceived ideas which subconsciously suggest the manner in which the movement or series of movements should be performed;

(3) The new and conscious mental orders which will set in motion the muscular mechanism essential to the correct performance of the action;

(4) The movements (contractions and expansions) of the muscles which carry out the mental orders. The process of re-education concerns itself with establishing these principles, and for the purpose of illustration we may take a typical example of a patient who has had no experience of them.

A well-built, muscular man in the prime of life, conducting during business hours a sedentary occupation and taking more or less violent exercise during his leisure, becomes a chronic sufferer from indigestion with all its concomitant troubles. He complains that the physical exercises of the gymnasium no longer do him any good, but appears to think that if he gave up his office work altogether—an economic impossibility for him—he might recover.

Suppose he is asked to stand upright and take a "deep breath." It will be found that he immediately makes movements which tend to retard the proper action of the respiratory processes rather than to promote such action. For instance, it is almost certain that in the attempt to make the movement referred to he will stiffen the muscles of his neck, throw back the head, hollow the back, protrude the stomach, and take breath by audibly *sucking* air into the lungs. The muscles over the entire surface of the bony thorax will be unduly tensed, tending to more or less harmful thoracic rigidity at the very moment when the maximum of mobility is needed. How could the result be otherwise? For, in telling the pupil to take a "deep breath," the teacher starts out with the assumption that the pupil can do so. But why such an assumption? What guide in carrying out the order has the pupil except his own admittedly erroneous guidance? I say "admittedly" erroneous, for I contend that the pupil's condition, together with the fact that he and the teacher deem it necessary to remedy it, is tantamount to this admission. So common, so almost universal is such a response as the above to these orders that the truth of the statement may be tested on any average individual. Now the mistakes of this response need not be dwelt upon here. They have proved in every case in my experience sufficient explanation for the trouble of the digestive organs. Examination of the subject will reveal the hollowing of the back with the accompanying protrusion of the abdominal wall, whilst the abdominal muscles will be deficient in the energy and tone necessary to the maintenance of efficiency in the digestive organs. Now in dealing with this case, many parts of the organism will require readjustment. The spine must be straightened and lengthened, the mean thoracic capacity permanently increased in order to give free play to the internal organs, and the firmly established habit of drawing breath by *sucking* air into the lungs must be broken.

It is essential in this place to point out that no system of physical exercises will alter the present condition of the subject in respect of these faults, since all exercises will be conducted under a primary misconception with regard to the use of the muscles involved in the readjustment and co-ordination of the organism.

We may now follow the individual through the four stages in the inculcation of the principles of conscious control. In the first place it is necessary that he should have a clear understanding of the faults we seek to remedy. No tacit compliance on his part to a treatment, the processes of which he does not understand, will be of the slightest value. He must accept completely the principle in detail. In the second place he must be taught to realize his erroneous conceptions which result in erroneous movements, and this, whether the conceptions be conscious or subconscious. He must also be taught to inhibit, and, finally, to eradicate these preconceived ideas and the mental order or series of orders which follow from them. Only then can he give the correct guiding orders as next described.

In the third place, then, he must learn to give the correct mental orders to the mechanisms involved, and *there must be a clear differentiation in his mind between the giving of the order and the performance of the act ordered and carried out through the medium of the muscles.* The whole principles of volition and inhibition are implicit in the recognition of this differentiation. Thus, to return to the example under consideration, we will suppose that I have requested the pupil *to order* the spine to lengthen and the neck to relax. If, instead of merely framing and holding this desire in his mind, he attempts the physical performance of these acts, he will invariably stiffen the muscles of his neck and shorten his spine, since these are the movements habitually associated *in his mind* with lengthening his spine, and the muscles will contract in accordance with the old associations. In effect it will be seen that in this, as in all other cases, stress must be laid on the point that it is *the means* and not the *end* which must be considered. When the end is held in mind, instinct or long habit will always seek to attain the end by habitual methods. The action is performed below the level of consciousness in its various stages, and only rises to the level of consciousness when the end is being attained by the correct "means whereby."

In the fourth place, when the correct guiding orders have been practised and given by the mind—a result attained by attention and the instruction of the teacher—the muscles involved will come into play in different combinations under the control of conscious guidance, and a reasoned act will take the place of the series of habitual, unconsidered movements which have resulted in the deformation of the body. And it must be kept clearly in mind that the whole of the old series of movements has been correlated and compacted into one indivisible and rigid sequence which has invariably followed the one mental order that started the train; such an order, for instance, as "Stand upright."

Leaving this specific example, I come now to a consideration of the general principles involved. Firstly, as to the teaching method.

Every one who has had experience, personally or vicariously, of the many "methods" and "systems" of teaching breathing, speaking, singing, physical-culture, golf, fencing, etc., must have noticed that whilst the failures of these "methods" are many, the successes are comparatively few.

The few successes are of course set down to exceptional natural aptitude, whilst the teacher has an explanation of those cases more flattering to himself and prefers not to consider too closely the average of his failures. The truth is that all these systems break down because the pupil, in the attempt to adopt them, is guided always by his subconscious direction and is forced to depend too much on what is called natural aptitude. When guidance by conscious control and reason supersedes guidance by instinct, we shall be able to develop our potentialities to the full.

My own analysis of the matter is that the teaching method is, as a rule, entirely wrong, and wrong because of a fundamental misconception and an entirely inaccurate analysis, resulting in a false premise. The pupil's defects are dealt with commonly through their effects and not their causes. It is not recognized that every defective action is the result of the erroneous preconception of the doer, whether consciously or subconsciously exercised, and the orders which directly or indirectly follow. Nor is it understood that a pupil under the influence of such erroneous preconceptions can make no real progress till he is made to realize that it is he himself who is actually bringing about the defective action. The teacher does not attach sufficient importance to the fact that the pupil is often under a complete misapprehension as to his own actions, being under the delusion that he is doing one thing when he is often doing the exact opposite.

No real progress in the overcoming of faults can be made until the pupil consciously ceases to will or to do those things which he has been willing and doing in the past, and which have led him to commit the faults that are to be eradicated. " Don't do this, but this," says the teacher, dealing with *effects*. In other words, it is assumed that the defective action on the part of the pupil can be put right by "doing something else." The teacher accepts and preaches this doctrine without ever analysing the defect to its root cause in the human will, the motor of the whole mechanism. He forgets that in "doing something else" the pupil must use the same machinery which, *ex hypothesi,* is working imperfectly, and that he must be guided in his action by the same erroneous conceptions regarding right and wrong doing. Neither teacher nor pupil seems to remember that to know whether practice is *right* or *wrong* demands judgment. Judgment is the result of experience. Faulty or wrong experience means faulty or bad judgment, whereas correct experience means good judgment.

The very fact that the pupil was beset with defects and needed help proves that his *kinaesthetic* experiences were incorrect and even harmful, and as his judgment on the kinaesthetic basis has been built upon such faulty experience, the judgment will prove most misleading and unsound.

Therefore we are forced to dispense, for the time being, with the sense of feeling as a guide in its old sphere of associations. We cannot deny that we are beset with defects, that even when the way is made clear for their eradication we cannot follow that way on our old mode of procedure, because our guides in the form of sensory appreciations (feeling-tones), general experience, and judgment are unworthy of our confidence, and will guide us in such a way that, even if we succeed in eradicating some specific defect, it will be found that in the process we have cultivated a number of others which are as bad or even worse than the original.

It seems also to me that practice so called is so rarely directed by a reasoned analysis on a reasoned plan. Nor does the teacher analyse and instruct with accuracy. He demands from the pupil merely imitative, not reasoned acts. This makes practice so often futile for the imperfectly co-ordinated person, and teaching both halting and inadequate.

With regard to this question of the imitative method I have frequently had to point out to vocal pupils that certain effects and capacities, which they hoped to acquire in a few lessons, were a result of a proper conscious knowledge on my part of the "means whereby" the voice is produced. To achieve these results they must study and master the same principles, but they could never reproduce them by a series of imitative acts divorced from knowledge of the processes involved and skill in using these processes. There is no royal road to anything worth having, and the imitative method of teaching seems to me pure charlatanry.

The position of the teacher and pupil is a very hopeless one as long as their standpoint is still on the subconscious plane, and the physical and mental conditions of our time, when considered in the light of the teaching methods adopted in the past, afford abundant proof of this.

My reader can rejoice that the foregoing is a faithful representation of our position to-day. He can rejoice because these tremendous forces demand that if he wishes to progress he must leave the subconscious plane of animal growth and development, and adopt the reasoned conscious plane of guidance and control by means of which mankind may rise to those high evolutionary planes for which his latent and undeveloped potentialities fit him.

I will now endeavour to outline the teaching method which should be adopted if we are to pass successfully from subconscious to conscious guidance and control, in the endeavour to remove defects and delusions and to develop and establish correct guiding centres and senses.

The conscious guidance and control advocated here is on a wide and general, and not on a specific basis. Conscious control applied in a specific way is unthinkable, except as a result of the principle primarily applied as a universal. For instance, the conscious controlling of the movements of a particular muscle or limb, as practised by athletes and others, is of little practical value in the science of living. The specific control of a finger, of the neck, or of the legs should primarily be the result of the conscious guidance and control of the mechanism of the torso, particularly of the antagonistic muscular actions which bring about those correct and greater co-ordinations intended to control the movements of the limbs, neck, respiratory mechanism, and the general activity of the internal organs.

In order to describe the teaching method necessary in this connection I will indicate the procedure which should be adopted in the attempt to help a pupil in whom undue tension of the muscles of one side of the neck causes the head to be pulled down on that side. In the ordinary way, the pupil is told to relax and straighten the neck and he and his teacher devote themselves to this end. This attempt may be attended with more or less success, chiefly less. If they do succeed in removing the specific trouble it is almost certain that new defects will have been cultivated during the process. In any case the teacher's order to relax and straighten the neck is incorrect and primarily the result of a wrong assumption. It started from a false premise which led to false deductions. The pupil and his teacher decided that something was wrong and that therefore something specific had to be done to put it right. The "end" was held in mind primarily and not the "means whereby."

The correct point of view is: Something is wrong in the use of the psycho-physical mechanism of the person concerned. Is this imperfection or defect a direct or indirect result of this person's own direction and action, or is it the result of some influence outside of himself and beyond his power to control? It can be proved conclusively that his imperfections or defects are due entirely to causes springing directly or indirectly from his own ideas and acts.

It is therefore obvious that the correct order of procedure for teacher and pupil is first for the pupil to learn to prevent himself from doing the wrong things which cause the imperfections or defects, and then, as a *secondary* consideration in procedure, to learn the correct way to use the mental and physical mechanisms concerned. If there is any undue muscular pull in any part of the neck, it is almost certain to be due to the defective co-ordination in the use of the muscles of the spine, back, and torso generally, the correction of which means the eradication of the real cause of the trouble.

This principle applies to the attempted eradication of all defects or imperfect uses of the mental and physical mechanisms in all the acts of daily life and in such games as cricket, football, billiards, baseball, golf, etc., and in the physical manipulation of the piano, violin, harp, and all such instruments.

My reader must not fail to remember that mental conceptions are the stimuli to the ideo-motor centre which passes on the subconscious or conscious guiding orders to the mechanism. In dealing with human defects or imperfections we must consider the inherited subconscious conceptions associated with the mechanisms involved, and also the conceptions which are to be the forerunners of the ideo-motor guiding orders connected with the new and correct use of the different mechanisms.

In order to establish successfully the latter (correct conception), we must first inhibit the former (incorrect conception), and from the ideo-motor centre project the new and different directing orders which are to influence the complexes involved, gradually eradicating the tendency to employ the incorrect ones, and steadily building up those which are correct and reliable.

It will therefore be understood that if we eliminate the conception established and associated with our defects or imperfections, it means that we are really eliminating our inherited subconsciousness, and all the defective uses of the psycho-physical mechanism connected therewith.

In our attempts on these lines we are, at the outset, confronted with the difficulty of mental rigidity. The preconceptions and habits of thought with regard to the uses of the muscular mechanisms are the first if not the only stumbling blocks to the teaching of conscious control. Many of these preconceptions are the legacy of instinct, others arise from habitual practices started by a faulty comprehension of the uses of the mechanism, others again by conscious or unconscious imitation of faults in others. In this last case it may be noted that although we are always deploring the degeneracy of civilized man, the exemplars held up for the child's conscious and unconscious imitation are nearly always faulty specimens. These preconceptions and habits of thought, therefore, must be broken down, and since the reactions of mind on body and body on mind are so intimate, it is often necessary to break down these preconceptions of mind by performing muscular acts for the subject vicariously; that is to say, the instructor must move the parts in question while the subject attends to the inhibition of all muscular movements. It would be impossible, however, to describe the method in full detail in this place, owing to the extraordinary variability of the cases presented, no two of which exhibit precisely the same defects. On broad lines it is evident that the misuses must be diagnosed by the instructor, who may be called upon to use considerable ingenuity and patience in correcting the faults, and substituting the correct mental orders for the one general order which starts the old train of vicious habitual movements. The mental habit must be first attacked, and this mental habit usually lies below the level of consciousness; but it may be reached by introspection and analysis, and by the performance of the habitual acts by other than the habitual methods— that is, by physical acts performed consciously as an effect of the conscious conception and the conscious direction of the mind.

Speaking generally, it will be found that the pupil is quite unable to analyse his own actions. Tell a young golfer that he has taken his eye off the ball or swayed his body, and he feels sure, in his heart, that you are mistaken. The imperfectly poised person has not a correct apprehension of what he is really doing. In this apparently simple matter of the carriage or poise of the body I find in quite nine-tenths of my cases a harmful rigidity[18] which is quite unconsciously assumed. When it is pointed out to them, and physically demonstrated, they almost invariably deny it indignantly. I ask a new pupil to put his shoulders back and his head forward, and he will consistently put both back or forward. I tell a new pupil he is shortening his spine, and in attempting to lengthen it he invariably shortens it still more. The action is one over which he has neither learnt nor practised any

---

[18] A very notable though trivial instance of mental "rigidity" was brought to me by a pupil while writing these pages. A fireman on duty at a theatre had neglected to unbolt the escape doors. When severely reprimanded he pleaded that he had been instructed by an assistant manager to do duty in another part of the theatre at the time he usually opened the escapes. The following night the assistant manager instructed him to make the same change in his routine, on which the man pleaded, "Don't ask me to do that, sir. I forgot the escapes last night and I am sure to forget 'em again if you make me go that way round. You see, sir, I've gone round the other way so long that if I make a change I seem to lose my memory."

control whatever. He is simply deluded regarding his sensations and unable to direct his actions. I do not therefore, in teaching him, actually order him to lengthen his spine by performing any explicit action, but I cause him to rehearse the correct guiding orders, and after placing him in a position of mechanical advantage I am able by my manipulation to bring about, directly or indirectly as the case may be, the desired flexibility and extension.

The process is of course repeated until the pupil gains a new kinaesthetic sense of the new and correct use of the parts, which become properly co-ordinated, and the correct habit is established. He will then no longer find it easy to cause his physical machinery to work as it did before the fault was thus effectively eradicated.

I frequently have to treat cases of congenital or acquired crippling and distortion. I protest against the mental attitude which looks upon such ailments as incurable and beyond the control of the patient— the mental attitude of the person who says, "Poor fellow," to the sufferer, and induces him to repeat and be dominated by this paralysing formula. As a matter of plain fact the condition is maintained by the pupil's erroneous ideas concerning "cause" and "effect," and the working of his own mechanism, and so, subconsciously but quite effectively, he is really causing and maintaining the trouble. My method is to make an examination and then to apply tests to discover the real cause or causes—namely, the erroneous preconceived ideas—and to find out what minimum of control is left, and therefrom to develop a healthy condition of the whole organism by a simple and practical procedure which step by step effects the desired physical and mental changes. Like the faithhealer, then, I lay much stress on the mental attitude of, the patient; unlike him, instead of denying the existence of the evil, I make the pupil search out with me its cause. I then explain to him that his own will (not mine or some higher will) is to effect the desired change, but that it must first be directed in a rational way to bring about a physical manifestation, and must be aided by a simple mechanical principle and a proper manipulation. In this way a reasoned and permanent confidence is built up in the pupil instead of a spurious hysterical one which is apt to fail as suddenly as it arose. I will not, for instance, allow my pupils to close their eyes during their work, in spite of a constant plea that they can "think better" or "concentrate" better with their eyes shut, for, as a rule, I find that this resolves itself into an attempt at self-hypnotism. I make them endeavour to exercise their conscious minds all the while. As I have already said, I maintain further, and I am prepared to prove, that the majority of physical defects have come about by the action of the patient's own will operating under the influence of erroneous preconceived ideas and consequent delusions, exercised consciously or, more often, subconsciously, and that these conditions can be changed by that same will directed by a right conception implanted by the teacher.

In this connection I am able to give particulars of an interesting case.

A well-known actor fell during rehearsal and injured his arm so severely that he was unable to raise it more than five or six inches from his side without intense pain. He consulted many medical men without relief, and had been disabled for six weeks when he was sent to see me.

I diagnosed the case as a subjective subconsciously willed disablement. Of course, the last thing I mean is that it was "affected" in the usual sense; all the patient's interests and character made this impossible.

I asked him to lift his arm. "I can't." "But please try." He did so, and the cause of his trouble was immediately apparent to me. He was using the muscular mechanisms of the arm and neck in such a way as to place a severe strain on the injured muscle, such a strain, indeed, as would have been harmful to a normal arm, and which caused him intense pain. For instance, he was exerting force sufficient to lift a sack of flour, and he *looked* as if he had been called upon for such an exertion! He was stiffening all the muscles which he should have relaxed, and was altogether acting as the subconsciously controlled person of to-day does habitually act when something unusual occurs. To put the matter in the terms of my thesis, he acted in accordance with a subconscious guiding influence which had long since lost the standard of accuracy of instinct possessed by his early ancestors, whilst nothing had been given to or cultivated by him in his civilized state to compensate for its loss. The "cure" was so simple as to appear ludicrous. I had diagnosed that the subconsciously stiffened muscles were the cause of the trouble. My efforts were devoted to obtaining the correct action of the arm with the minimum of tension. This was done by manipulation and by giving him guiding orders which brought about the correct use of the parts concerned. Within ten minutes he was able to lift his arm with very little pain and he resumed his professional work at once and without relapse. Note that the relaxing was not brought about by a preliminary order to relax, an action which entailed processes of which he had no true consciousness and over which therefore he had no control. Note also that this demonstration is much more effective for the treatment of similar later accidents and for general self-development and control, than any hypnotic "suggestion" that there was no pain.[19]

I do not deny, for it would be against the evidence, that the healers do contrive to remove pain; but apart from the danger of removing mere symptoms (that is, removing nature's danger signals and leaving the danger untouched), their methods have the obvious limitation of being repugnant to many, and have fallen into some discredit among those who are by no means among the least capable, accomplished, and thoughtful human types.

Another very interesting case was that of a man who stuttered and came to me for help. All stutterers have their particular and peculiar little accompaniments to the main defect. His was a harmful habit of moving his arm up and down from the elbow as he attempted to

---

[19] "This experimental observation is so far to our interest that it has proved that hypnotic suggestion is by far surpassed in the duration of its effects by suggestion in the waking state, and this again by regular teaching and practice. But this is physiologically explicable: Hypnotic suggestion obtains its results solely through the intensity of the isolated stimulus and through the brain-track it leaves behind, which has an abnormally slight connection with the whole associative mechanism of the brain. Regular instruction, on the contrary, is based on the strong associative implanting of the stimulus and the brain-track it leaves behind, with the normal activity of the brain, i.e., on the many-sidedness of the nervous connections and their reproductive effect; whilst in the first case the trace is more or less easily effaced, in the second the accompanying reproductive, sympathetic stimulus increases and preserves the result obtained, as well as effecting the other bodily functions dependent on it."—*The Psychic Treatment of Disease,* Berthold Kern.

speak. I asked him why he did this, and he replied that he *felt* it assisted him in speaking. I explained and demonstrated to him that this was a delusion, that this movement of the limb was really a hindrance and not an assistance. He saw that a considerable amount of valuable mental and physical energy, which should have been conveyed to the mechanisms and organs of speech, was being diverted to a limb which might have been amputated without interfering in any way with those mental and mechanical processes on which his powers of speech entirely depended. He became convinced on these points and intimated his willingness to endeavour to carry out my instructions. I assisted him to establish a working conscious control basis and improved his co-ordination generally.

Then I made the following request:

"I wish you to project orders to these newly developed co-ordinators. You will then be prevented from employing your arms as an aid in speaking, and in your general attempts at conscious guidance in private. In public I wish you to adopt the following mode of procedure:

"Whenever a person speaks to you, asking a question or in any way trying to open up a conversation, you must as a primary principle refuse to answer by mentally saying *No*. (This will hold in check the old subconscious orders— the bad habit of moving the arm. It constitutes the inhibition of the old errors before attempting to speak.)

"Then give the new and correct orders to your general co-ordinations and command the ' means whereby' of the act of correct and controlled speaking.

"Make this a principle of life."

Perhaps I should add here that I convinced this pupil by practical demonstrations that the energy directed to his arm was wasted and misdirected; that, if this energy were correctly directed to the proper co-ordinations concerned with the mechanism of breathing and speaking, the process would represent the difference between correct and incorrect attempts in the direction of ultimate satisfactory breath and speech control. In this particular case the desired end was gained in a few weeks.

The observant person must have noted the singularly small range of physical control exercised by the average adult outside the narrow sphere of his daily routine actions. In the realm of sport, for instance, take the golf swing. A novice, or for that matter a player of some experience, carefully "addresses" the ball and is instructed *to swing up and down again in the same orbit,* without moving the head or swinging the body. The professional has arranged that stance; the drive seems the simplest of actions; yet, more often than not, it fails lamentably. And the player, nine times out of ten, *has no sort of consciousness* of what has interfered with his stroke.

This is a very common instance of the failure to achieve the desired end in those who depend solely on subconscious direction. Even the accomplished and practised golfer has periods when he acknowledges that he is "off his game" or "out of form," times when his skill leaves him altogether *because he cannot register consciously* the method which, when he uses it instinctively, enables him to play well.

Where the novice is concerned, however, the stubborn fact to be faced is that it is practically impossible for the ordinary person to, carry out such instructions as *swing up and down again in the same orbit, etc.,* with precision and accuracy. At the first attempt the pupil may, by mere chance, succeed. He may even make a second successful attempt, and a third, and so on. But such instances are very rare. On the other hand, he may begin badly and after a few days record a series of successes. Incidentally, I will point out that this applies more or less to the majority of experienced golf players. We all know that to vary is to be human. But there should not be such an alarming gulf between our best and our worst. It is very serious from the mental point of view. It shakes our confidence in ourselves to the very roots of our mental and physical foundations. Such experiences have a bad effect even upon the emotions generally, and the person concerned develops irritation, bad temper, and other undesirable traits at a time (a time of recreation and pleasure) when there should be an absolute absence of these harmful conditions.

It will readily be conceded that during our attempts at this or any other game the mental condition of the performer should be in keeping with a pleasurable and health-giving form of outdoor exercise.

But to return to the stumbling-blocks in the way of the correct performance of an act which requires one "to swing up and down in the same orbit." These arise mainly from the tendency of the great majority to curve and shorten the spine unduly and otherwise to interfere with the correct conditions of the muscular system of the back, the spine, and the thorax in the performance of certain physical acts.[20] These tendencies are particularly marked when the arms are employed in such a movement as the "swing down" to make the stroke following the preparatory "swing up." Consequently not one person in a thousand is capable of maintaining during the *down* stroke those conditions of the back and spine present during the *up* stroke. Consideration of these points will indicate that in order "to swing up and down in the same orbit," it is essential that the position of the spine—particularly as regards its length and relative poise during the up and down movement—:must be maintained. Other conditions are of course necessary, but I cannot deal with more than one or two of the chief factors.

In order to secure the proper use of the arms and legs, correct mental guidance and control are necessary. Such guidance and control should, of course, be conscious. Furthermore, this mental guidance and control must co-ordinate with a proper position and length of the spine and the accompanying correct muscular uses of the torso, if these limbs are to be controlled by that guidance and co-ordination which will command their accurate employment at all times within reasonable limits.

The foregoing are a few of the fundamental difficulties with which the golf teacher and pupil are beset. Those who have taken lessons will at once admit that the ordinary teaching methods fail to reach these difficulties satisfactorily. As a matter of fact they are not even taken

---

[20] [1] A simple experiment will serve to prove this shortening by the increase of, say, the lumbar curve. Take a piece of cardboard of six inches in length and place it flat on a table or against the wall. With a pencil draw lines on the table or wall as close to the upper and lower ends of the cardboard as possible. Remove the cardboard and curve it slightly across the lower portion about an inch from the end which touched the lowest line. Replace it on the lower line without interfering with the curve, and you will find that it does not reach the upper line any longer. A similar condition occurring in the human being means a shortening in stature.

into consideration. The orthodox teaching method holds the "end" in view and not the "means whereby." It depends on the giving of orders on the "end-gaining" principle—such an order, for instance, as "Swing up and down again in the same orbit," without consideration of the "means whereby"; that is, without making certain that the pupil has the power to maintain a proper position of his spine and back and to use the limbs correctly during the performance of such physical acts. In other words, the teacher should first discover if his pupil is reasonably correctly co-ordinated in those muscular uses of his organism which are essential to the proper carrying out of instructions necessary to the performance of definite physical acts demanding co-ordination in the use of the human body and limbs.

If these tests are not made, the beginner will waste much valuable time, dissipate his energies, suffer needless worry and suspense, and become unduly apprehensive in his attempt to gain even a very moderate standard of dependable excellence in playing golf or other games to which he may devote himself. If we employ as the fundamental in teaching the principles of conscious guidance and control on a basis of re-education and general co-ordination the following advantages should accrue:

(1) The pupil will be made aware of his specific defects in the employment of his mental and physical organism in physical performances.

(2) When he has been made aware of these defects, he can be taught to inhibit the faulty movements, and his teacher can assist him to gain slowly but correctly the necessary experiences in the correct use of those muscular mechanisms which will enable him sooner or later to govern them properly without the aid of the teacher, and to employ them with accuracy and precision in his game of golf and other physical performances.

(3) In the golf act under consideration he must first be given the correct experiences in the use of the muscular mechanisms of the torso and legs with the arms falling naturally at his side.

(4) The correct experiences should then be given with the use of the arms in making the "up stroke." When this act can be performed without interference with the satisfactory

conditions of the torso and legs, the correct experiences should be given in making the "down stroke," but without attempting to *drive* the ball. This latter portion of the whole act should not be attempted until the pupil is familiar with the different movements described in 1, 2, 3, and 4.

(5) When the attempt to drive is finally made, the idea to be held in mind is that of *repeating the experiences as a whole* (in other words, the "means whereby"), not the idea of making a drive. If the pupil holds the "end" (i.e., making a drive) in mind he will at once revert to all his old subconscious habits in the use of his mental and physical organism, whereas, on the other hand, if he holds in mind the "means whereby" (his new correct experiences), he will sooner or later put them correctly into practice and make his drives with an accuracy and precision which will give the maximum of satisfaction and pleasure.

I have personal knowledge of a person who, by employing the principles of conscious control which I advocate, mounted and rode a bicycle downhill without mishap on the first attempt, and on the second day rode 30 miles out and 30 miles back through normal traffic. This same person was also able to fence passably on first taking the foil into his hands. In each case the principles involved were explained to him and he carefully watched an exhibition, first analysing the actions and the "means whereby," then reproducing them on a clearly apprehended plan. This, it seems to me, should be a normal, not an abnormal human accomplishment. Just as a cat by sheer instinct, the first time she essays to jump, gauges her powers and the distances with accuracy, so, with more reason and greater ease, the human subject, by employing consciously controlled intellect and kindred experience in place of instinct, should be able to direct his powers to a definite ordained end with less physical strain and less frequent physical repetition, i.e., "Practice."

In this connection I have been often asked the difference between instinct and intuition. I define instinct as the result of the accumulated subconscious psycho-physical experiences of man at all stages of his development, which continue with us until, singly or collectively, we reach the stage of conscious control; whilst intuition is the result of the *conscious reasoned* psycho-physical experiences during the process of our evolution. The word "subconsciousness" is but a formula for our habits of life. I hold strongly that when we shall have reached the state of conscious control in civilization, and have established thereby new and correct habits, a new and correct subconscious-ness will become established.

I might here with advantage re-emphasize my view regarding the supreme importance of conscious control.

Conscious control is imperative, as I have pointed out, because instinct in our advancing civilization largely fails to meet the needs of our complex environment. Without conscious control the subject or patient may know he has defects, may know further what those defects are, may even know at what explicit improvement he is to aim, and yet may be quite unable by means of imitation or the orthodox and traditional methods of instruction to effect the desired end.

With conscious control, on the other hand, true development (unfolding), education (drawing out), and evolution are possible along intellectual as against the old orthodox and fallacious lines, by means of reasoned processes, analysed, understood, and explicitly directed. Conscious control enables the subject, once a fault be recognized, to find and readily apply the remedial process.

It is my belief, confirmed by the research and practice of nearly twenty years, that man's supreme inheritance of conscious guidance and control is within the grasp of any one who will take the trouble to cultivate it. That it is no esoteric doctrine or mystical cult, but a synthesis of entirely reasonable propositions that can be demonstrated in pure theory and substantiated in common practice.

I will now consider at greater length a characteristic case for the elucidation of these various points of theory and practice.

H., a youth fourteen years old, was sent to me by a wellknown throat specialist. He had removed two nodules from the boy's vocal cords, and had given him special treatment in a nursing home for a month, but without any satisfactory improvement. The mother came to me with the boy and was present during my treatment. I found that his attempts to speak resulted in a hoarse whisper accompanied by spasmodic twitchings of various parts of the body and by facial contortions, all this being brought about by erroneous conceptions, left untouched by the former teacher, as to the amount of effort needed in order to speak. In his former lessons he had been told to try to improve the utterance of simple sounds and words, without any analysis or pointing out of the wrong means which he had previously employed to this end. All his efforts to carry out his teacher's directions were made in accordance with his original preconceptions and former experience. His muscular mechanisms were employed in the same (wrong) way, and his whole consciousness and explicit and implicit self-directions were exactly the same as they had been previously.

He had opened his mouth imperfectly and had been ordered by his teacher to open his mouth wider. But there had been no recognition by the pupil that he had not opened his mouth sufficiently, neither had there been any analysis by the teacher of the pupil's failure to open the mouth (a seemingly simple thing but *ex hypothesi* not simple to the patient), or of the concomitant contortions and automatic reaction. As well say, "You have been speaking improperly, now speak properly," and call that a lesson, as indeed it would have been called in the early Victorian era, as, "Open your mouth wide, speak up, and don't make nervous movements." It is not the "end" that the teacher and pupil must work for, but the "means whereby." And this discovery of the "means whereby," differing in different subjects and not to be stated in a general formula, can only be the result of trained observation and careful, patient investigation and experience. In practice, the anxiety of this particular pupil to *speak* long the lines of his old preconceived ideas, when nothing had been done to remove them, had made his many lessons fruitless, and had set in motion the old habitual train of irrelevant and hampering actions.

My own treatment, then, is: First to observe and analyse and bring about a proper working of the machinery in general (nature does not work in parts but as a whole) ; then to point out the first guiding order or orders to be brought into play by the pupil—namely, the inhibiting of the tension of the muscles working the lower jaw. The pupil must be made to realize clearly that this involves no action whatever on his part, but that he need only remember the correct inhibiting orders and employ them in accordance with definite instructions.

When he does this it at once results in the freeing of his jaw, enabling me to move it for him with my hand. This gives him for the first time the correct kinsesthetic sense in connection with the action of his jaw and makes it clear once and for all to him that the desired action is perfectly and easily possible.

The subconscious jerkings and contortions pointed out one by one are patiently inhibited by the pupil, sometimes directly, but more often by the explicit use, under my direction, of guiding orders which gradually co-ordinate and remedy the whole faulty system* of the pupil's muscular action.   One by one the wrong actions and reactions are inhibited, the tightening of the neck, the throwing back of the head, the tension of the lower jaw, the deep "sucking" breath, the jerks of the limbs, the grimaces; and then, on the positive side, the right actions are gradually built up, such as the free controlled opening of the mouth, the even "pneumatic" breath, the upright balanced poise, the clear enunciation and correct vocalization. [21]

The brain of both pupil and teacher are at work the whole time. No use is made of "hypnotism" or of auto-suggestion, but the confident, skilful, patient, and explicit directions of the teacher should tend to remove flurry and vagueness and consequent waste of mental and physical effort.

The analysis of even the simplest processes is apt to appear unduly complex. This case can be stated briefly on the practical side. It took twenty lessons to break down the bad habits and another twelve to effect a complete and permanent cure.

With regard to such a simple act as opening the mouth two or three factors should be emphasized: firstly, the tendency to yield to erroneous preconceived ideas; secondly, the delusions of the pupil in regard to thought and action; thirdly a pernicious dependence on sensation which has been based solely upon experience of defective action.

There are very few men, for instance, who, when told to open the mouth, will not throw the head back with the idea, as it were, of lifting the upper jaw away from the lower. They do not observe or

---

[21] As I have already explained in Part I, inspiration is not a sucking of air into the lungs but an inevitable instantaneous rush of air into the partial vacuum caused by the automatic expansion of the thorax.

reflect that an inhibition of the subconscious orders which cause the mechanisms to keep the mouth closed will bring about such a relaxation of that muscular tension as will allow the jaw to drop. It does in fact commonly drop in the case of that type of idiot who is most often open-mouthed ; whilst it is common knowledge that in boxing a blow on the head, heavy enough to throw out the controlling gear, causes the jaw of the injured boxer to drop of itself and to remain dropped for a considerable time.

When I ask a pupil to let me move his lower jaw away from his upper he usually increases instinctively the tension that keeps the lower jaw in place. As I have frequently pointed out, an enormous aggregate waste of energy is involved in these constant and irrational tensions.

But the matter becomes seriously harmful in, let us say, such actions as singing and speaking, for when the mouth is opened with this unconscious and absurd expenditure of force, the neck is unduly stiffened, the head is thrown backwards, the larynx unduly and harmfully depressed, and thereby in a position most unfavourable to good vocalization. As I have for years pointed out and demonstrated in my own practice, from these ill-considered tensions spring the different forms of throat and ear trouble which are so common and which so frequently defy ordinary or for that matter extraordinary and highly specialized medical treatment. By inducing a proper conception of the right method of opening the mouth, I can command in the patient, and, what is more important, teach him to command in himself, a free condition in which the larynx tends to be slightly raised and relaxed instead of tightened and depressed; whilst there will surely follow, and that with a minimum of effort, a greater mobility of the facial muscles and of those of the lips and tongue so essential to good and clear enunciation and vocalization.

This, in the briefest summary, is the method of teaching the process of conscious control of the muscular mechanisms. I come now to an equally brief consideration of the effects of this method. Speaking generally, I have found that the first immediate effects are a general stimulation and increased efficiency of the whole organism. Nor is this difficult to understand. For it would seem that in the life led by civilized man so little demand is made upon any but the commonly exercised muscles, and these are called upon for comparatively so little effort, that a general sluggishness supervenes, with consequent stagnation resulting in the commonly observed effects of autointoxication. With the breaking up of the old motor habits, the muscular mechanisms are brought into full play, the toxins which have accumulated are broken up and disturbed, and increased vitality, a sense of power, and enormously improved efficiency follow as a matter of course. Beyond this, and still speaking generally, I find that there are increased powers of resistance against the attacks of infectious diseases, and—possibly the greatest effect, since it guarantees the lasting qualities of the change which is brought about—an ability to check the formation of any bad, incipient muscular or mental habit. This last is, in my opinion, of the very first importance, for it demonstrates the power of the individual, once these principles of conscious guidance and control are mastered, to be the lord of his own body.

Of the specific effects procured by the inculcation of these methods I cannot speak at length, but I am able to produce a list of pupils who have been helped by me, and I have often been astonished by the results.

These include cases diagnosed by prominent physicians in England, Australia, and the United States of America as paralysis, varicosity, tuberculosis, asthma, adhesions of the lungs, haemorrhage, congenital and other malformations, effects of infantile paralysis, many varieties of throat, nose, and ear trouble, hay-fever, chronic constipation, incipient appendicitis, and colitis; and in no case that has come under , my personal supervision have I discovered any relapse that was not curable by a few further instructions in the principles enunciated.

Looking to the future and to the development and elaboration of this method, I foresee that a race which has been educated on the lines of what I have called "conscious guidance and control" will be eminently well fitted to meet any circumstance which the civilizations of the future may impose.

The minds and bodies alike of such a race will be adaptable to any occupation that may be their lot.

To those who have been educated in these principles no severe physical exercise is a necessity, since there are no stagnant eddies in the system in which the toxins can accumulate, and to them will belong a full and complete command of their physical organisms.

Matthias Alexander

That this practical and by no means visionary or untried psychotherapy will in time supersede the tentative and restricted methods of somato-therapy, I am confident, and I sincerely hope that the great benefits which these principles confer will not be confined to any one race or people. The wonderful improvements in physical health—often deemed "miraculous" by the uninitiated—which have been effected in adults, adumbrate the potentialities for efficiency which may be developed in the children of the new race.

It is essential that the peoples of civilization should comprehend the value of their inheritance, that outcome of the long process of evolution which will enable them to govern the uses of their own physical mechanisms. By and through consciousness and the application of a reasoning intelligence, man may rise above the powers of all disease and physical disabilities. This triumph is not to be won in sleep, in trance, in submission, in paralysis, or in anaesthesia, but in a clear, open-eyed, reasoning, deliberate consciousness and apprehension of the wonderful potentialities possessed by mankind, the transcendent inheritance of a conscious mind.

CHAPTER IV - CONSCIOUS GUIDANCE AND CONTROL IN PRACTICE

WHILST under the guidance of the subconscious mind, mankind cannot readily adapt itself to the rapidly and ever-changing conditions imposed by civilization. A proper standard of mental and physical perfection implies an adaptability which makes it easy for a man to turn from one occupation in which a certain set of muscles are employed, to another involving totally different muscular actions. Under the present subconscious guidance such an easy transference is, to say the least of it, likely to be a very rare occurrence.

For the purpose of demonstration we may assume that a man who has been engaged in clerical work all his life is suddenly called upon to become a ploughman and to make a success, within a reasonable time, of his new occupation.   This is an extreme instance, but the argument will apply equally well in a less extreme case. As he is subconsciously controlled he will attack the problem through his sense of feeling—through his feeling-tones—and strive directly for the desired "end."

He will make no reasoned estimate of the "means whereby" he may make a success.

He will not, as a preliminary to the act of ploughing, consider the particular demands which will be made on different parts of his organism, nor will he take into account the elemental laws which are essential to a satisfactory use of the plough as an instrument to be controlled in its legitimate sphere.

His mind is fixed from the start on the I achievement—on the act of ploughing.

He looks only to the end he desires to attain.

So he will grip the handles of his plough, set the horses in motion, and will be pleased to find that the plough moves more or less through the earth, chiefly less, for he finds it difficult to keep the share embedded and to keep the furrow straight. When he succeeds, he is almost certain to be thrown from side to side by the movements of the plough, which are affected by the hard or soft ground it meets in its progress. He holds no conscious reasoned guiding principles in his mind. His efforts are simply subconscious, in a chance endeavour to gain the end in view.

In order to maintain his own equilibrium and the efficient working of the plough, it is highly probable that he will unduly tense muscles which are precisely those which should not be tensed, and relax those which should do the most work. The tension of the muscles of the arm will almost certainly be unnecessarily high, and the general use of the wrong muscles will tend to destroy the proper equilibrium rather than to; maintain it. We thus see that the moment he steps into his new occupation (which he no doubt had congratulated himself would bring perfect health in its train), he immediately begins to cultivate new and harmful habits during his daily round. He becomes a badly co-ordinated, imperfectly guided ploughman precisely as he was a badly co-ordinated and imperfectly guided clerk. When the principles of reasoned conscious control are adopted, the man leading a sedentary life will be able to take up the occupation of ploughman without any fear of cultivating harmful habits. Moreover, he will attain proficiency in ploughing in one-tenth part of the time that the subconsciously controlled man took to obtain a half-mastery of it.

Let us see how he would set about it from the point of view of reasoned conscious guidance and control. Acting under the guiding principles of reasoned and conscious control, he will consider first the "means whereby" he may achieve his object, rather than that object itself. He will take time to consider well the factors to be overcome. It will be obvious to any one who will take the trouble to watch another man at the plough, that a great deal of proper manipulation is necessary to keep the share embedded and a straight furrow. The manipulation requires firstly the maintenance of the ploughman's equilibrium in very difficult circumstances. This consideration will make it clear to him that his body must remain comparatively steady and support the arms and legs as the trunk of a tree does its limbs, following as nearly perpendicularly as possible the line the furrow should take. It will be evident to him that the "give and take" of the joints of the arms and legs are the chief moving factors which should meet the different movements of the handles of the plough. His highly trained guiding sensations will not permit him to make more physical tension with any part of the muscular system than is absolutely necessary, and only the particular muscles best adapted for the control of his equilibrium and his plough will be called into special use. For instance, when the left handle of the plough is forced upwards and the right downwards by the plough being thrown into a position leaning towards the right, the ploughman's left arm will bend at the wrist, elbow, and shoulder, and the right straighten in order to maintain his equilibrium and general control without undue strain and interference with the proper position of the torso. Of course the left arm should exercise a downward pressure on the left handle, and the right should tend to pull the right handle upwards in order to straighten the plough again in its most effective position in the furrow. The left leg should be slightly bent at the knee, and the right leg should be kept straight and firm. The ploughman would thereby exercise his maximum of control in the right direction with the minimum of effort, and freedom from harmful strain. It will be clear from this example that in the consciously controlled stage of psycho-physical development men and women will be able, without fear of mental or physical harm, to adapt themselves at once to any strange or unusual circumstance in which they are placed. They will act in the face of the unaccustomed or the unsuspected at the direction of their conscious reasoning minds, before any promptings springing from the subconscious mind can take possession of them. Just as they will be able by conscious reasoning to change their habits at will, to be to-day a clerk, to-morrow a reasoning ploughman, so they will meet sudden surprise by that same conscious reasoning and accurate judgment which follows it. I have already drawn attention to the conduct of animals and of men and women in the lower stages of evolution when they are confronted with any phenomena to which they are unaccustomed; how that they stand terror-struck and immovable, and betray themselves. Such a condition of mind contains no element of control or reasoning, and the high importance of re-educating civilized men and women to a condition in which the control and reason are the main factors need scarcely be emphasized at this point. On all sides are seen the destruction, the waste, the loss in human lives and human energy which are the direct outcome of a civilization based on subconscious action.

It is our duty now to superimpose a new civilization founded on reason rather than on feeling-tones and debauched emotions, on conscious guidance and control rather than upon instinct. The savage is terror-struck when an eclipse passes over the sun; he bows to wood and stone, quivering with fear at any desecration of any of his puppet gods. Anything which has no place in his limited range of experience he approaches through instinct, which may preserve, but is more likely to betray him. To-day the greater part of mankind carries out the normal responsibilities of a lifetime guided by the same imperfect forces. Men have learnt the meaning of many things which to the savage were inscrutable, but when faced with the unknown they betray the same lack of control. Suddenly-angered men will make a retort which in the light of reflection appears to them foolish and inadequate. It is an everyday experience. In the calmer moments that follow they think of the "things they might have said," the things they might have done, which is a simple indication of the fact that in the heated moment their emotions held sway over them, whilst their reason and control were in abeyance. The subconsciously controlled person is immediately thrown into a state of panic when faced by any emergency which presents an element of danger.

In such circumstances many become self-hypnotic, and in this state will be found absolutely out of communication with their reason. As an instance of this, one may quote the behaviour of unbalanced people in a fire. In trying to save some of their possessions before making their escape they will as likely as not throw from the windows articles which will certainly be broken to atoms in their fall. The man who threw the drawing-room clock through the window and carried the hearth-rug downstairs is no fictional figure. His action represents the kind of behaviour that may be expected from the uncontrolled person in such an emergency. The following instance from my own experience may prove interesting in this connection.

I arrived late one evening at a large hotel in a well-known mining town in one of the Colonies. I was told that there was not a room available, but that if I cared to share a room with two beds in it, with two little sons of the proprietor, I might have a night's rest. Those who have any experience of a mining town where there is a "gold rush" on will appreciate my good fortune. Eight weary souls that night slept on the billiard-table and I do not remember how many found a bed on the hard, draughty floor of that same room. A great friend of mine was living at the hotel. He was a man of considerable learning and accounted by all who knew him as a fine scholar and the possessor of a fine intellect. The last injunction we received from the proprietor before he retired was, "Be sure to lock your door."

After a long chat with my friend we went very late to bed. Remembering the request of my host, I bolted the door, extinguished the light/and almost immediately fell into a sound sleep. Within an hour I was awakened by the crackling sound of burning wood and the roar of flames. I realized at once that the hotel was on fire, and almost immediately the tongues of flame found their way into my room through the top of the wooden walls and began to lick the ceiling of the bedroom.

My first thought was for the little lads who were sleeping in the room. I unbolted the door, and taking one under my left arm began to search for the other. By this time the room was filled with smoke, so I took the one boy out and returned to the search in the dense smoke. He had evidently jumped out of his bed half awake, for I found him under the bed. Taking both under my arms, I rushed down the stairs and ran with them to their father's bedroom. He dashed out and calling his menservants at once proceeded to take measures to extinguish the fire. I, of course, rushed to my friend's room, awakened him, and after lighting his candle and seeing him jump to the floor, I left him, and proceeded to give the general alarm. I then joined those who were fighting the flames, which after a while were successfully extinguished. My readers will be able from this account to judge of the time which elapsed between the visit to my friend's room and the complete extinguishing of the fire. When all was over I looked around to exchange a word with my friend, and was surprised to find that he was not of the number by whom we were surrounded. I walked back to his room, and was amazed to find him absolutely dressed. When I entered the room he was calmly buttoning up his waistcoat as on any other morning when he had nothing to fear. He was self-hypnotized as regarded his chances of being burned alive, and had even shaved.

Thousands of instances of similar behaviour in unusual circumstances might be given, and the list might well be completed with the now famous story concerning Carlyle's failure to keep in "communication with his reason" on the occasion that Henry Taylor was ill. He heard the news, and became over-anxious to help his friend. We can only conclude that he was under the domination of his sub-consciousness when he rushed off to Sheen with the remaining portion of a bottle of medicine which had helped Mrs. Carlyle, without knowing the particular uses of the medicine or the cause of his friend's illness.

The managing director of one of the largest business houses operating in Great Britain and America had been sent to me for treatment by his medical adviser. We had frequently discussed the psychological tendencies and characteristics of young men likely to make their way in the business world. One day, after a chat on this subject in which we were both interested, he informed me that there was always room in his firm for the right kind of young man, and intimated that if I knew one he would be glad if I would send him along. For some weeks prior to this time I had been asked to interest myself in a young man I had never met. I mentioned this to my pupil, and he said, "Ask the young man to write to me and I will fix an appointment." This was done, and the following is the young man's account of the interview:

"I called on Mr.... .and he positively insulted me.

When I entered his office he asked me to sit down while he finished a letter.

After about five minutes he jumped suddenly from his chair, walked towards me, and banging his fist with great vigour on a table near me, shouted, 'What the devil do you know about business?'

Of course, the young man continued, "I was so unnerved that I could not even collect my thoughts and I was so flurried that I could not answer his further questions. He told me he hadn't any position to suit me."

"My dear young man," I remarked, "why did you allow Mr....to insult you? Why did you not remonstrate with him and assure him that you could not permit him to speak to you in such a way?"

"I was so upset by his sudden attack, and I didn't expect to be treated in such a way."

"Just so," I replied, "you were nonplussed by the unexpected. But I hope this will be a lesson to you. Mr.... was only testing you, and he wants men who are capable of dealing with unexpected events and situations in his business. If you had made an instant protest against his manner, you would now be in a position in his firm because you would have come successfully through his test."

In that stage of evolution which may be defined as purely

animal, the powers of instinct in accustomed circumstances are quite remarkable, and it is due to that fact that the animal, in certain conditions of danger, will do the one right thing to escape. On the other hand, in proof of the limitations of instinct, we have only to name the noble and subconsciously controlled ostrich, so wily in its movements, and so clever in many directions, which, when confronted with more than an ordinary danger, presses its head into the sand and allows its pursuer to kill it. The powers of instinct are undoubtedly limited in the animal kingdom, in uncivilized mankind, and in all stages of evolution where subconscious control is the guiding principle. This fact perhaps accounts more than anything else for the rise and fall of nations and of races, for no community as yet has cultivated and developed a national consciousness in communication with reason. The psychology of nations is too large a subject to deal with here, but, logically, if the principles of conscious guidance and control, as I have outlined them in application to the individual, were further adopted by the rising nation, it is unthinkable that it should ever suffer from deterioration.

It would act in all crises strictly in accordance with the dictates of reason, and, guided by a judgment born of tested experience, it would be supreme.

CHAPTER V - CONSCIOUS GUIDANCE AND CONTROL

APPREHENSION AND RE-EDUCATION

THE average person may exhibit complete nerve control and balance during accustomed experiences and accomplishment of the different mental and physical demands made during the ordinary round of life, but when suddenly confronted with the unexpected or unknown he betrays undue apprehension and loss of control, even when the new experience may not hold any real terrors for him. The fact is, he becomes panic-stricken by the effects of the new experience. He is mentally incapable of considering the "facts of the case," for his reasoning power is thrown completely out of use by the unusual, and he is reduced to the level of the terrified animal or savage. This shows that we have not reached the stage of evolution where, by employing the reasoning faculties, we should be able to meet any emergency with control and calmness and do the right thing at the psychological moment. The really clever barrister takes advantage of this human weakness, and when cross-examining proceeds to unbalance the witness by an unexpected attack on a new line. If the barrister is successful in his choice in this connection he will assuredly gain his end with the witness who has not learnt to meet the unusual with reasoned judgment. He will become unnerved, and the barrister can hardly fail to succeed in disconcerting him.

Let me point out, however, that the barrister himself can be caught in the same trap if the witness adopts a mode of procedure which will be new to his rival. It will be merely a matter of which gets his blow in first. As an instance, in a case of special interest at which I was present, the following took place. Incidentally I should mention that the barrister and witness had a mutual friend by whom they had sent uncomplimentary messages to one another before the meeting in court. Naturally both were on guard. The barrister opened by, "Now, Mr...., might I suggest" and made the unfortunate mistake of repeating this the second time, whereupon the witness calmly remarked, "May I remind you that you are here to ask questions, not to suggest." The barrister was quite nonplussed for the moment. This disturbed his usual control and allowed his feelings to dominate his judgment, and during the remainder of the case he failed to regain his balance, and gave so much attention to trying to get even with the witness that he missed many points of the greatest value to his case and the verdict was gained by his opponents.

The removal of the Hunt Club Cup from its stand at Ascot Race Course is a trenchant example of the practical application of the knowledge of the weakness of men and women in the direction indicated. Constables and employees of the makers of the cup were on duty to ensure its safety and, moreover, there were always crowds of people round it. To any ordinary person it would have seemed absolutely impossible to remove such a large article without being detected. Despite this fact it was taken from its stand and removed from the Ascot grounds. One of those who successfully carried out this scheme must have been a highly developed psychologist, a man who knew only too well the weaknesses of his fellow-men. Presumably he knew that something unexpected must be done suddenly in order to attract and divert for a considerable length of time the constables guarding the Cup, during which time the thief would be enabled to get some distance away with his prize before its removal would be noticed. We are told that a group of men caused a disturbance, that heated words were exchanged and blows followed, no doubt at a prearranged signal. The thief counted on the psychological fact that the constables were unlikely to use their reason, and so preserve their self-control by continuing to watch the Cup in the face of this unexpected occurrence, and during the distraction therefore the theft was accomplished.

It must be obvious that there is going on a wicked waste of this wonderful power of reasoning, where reliance is placed on an automatic subconsciousness which permits the suspension of our common-sense and upsets our balance, thus narrowing our sphere of usefulness. Therefore, if we are really to progress in the future, subconscious guidance must be superseded by a reasoned and conscious guidance which can safeguard us in unusual circumstances and at critical moments. For with real progress on a sound basis we must expect a great increase in "critical moments" and "unusual circumstances," and our development must be on those lines which will enable us to meet them with calmness and common-sense, doing the one right thing the latter will suggest. This failing in reasoned action is as common among the educated as among the uneducated, and it is a most serious indictment of our present educational system that it should be so, and that as it is at present constituted it does not offer any real solution of the problem to be applied by the men and women of the future.

Take as an example a very prevalent form of human weakness — namely, our attitude of mind in regard to simple worries, whether real or imaginary. It is an interesting psychological fact that there are millions of highly educated people who have cultivated unwillingly what may be called the "worry habit." This worry habit is directly the outcome of the lack of use of our reasoning faculties, as is conclusively proved to me in my long professional experience by the fact that people suffering in this way worry exactly in the same degree when the cause has been removed as when it was actually a reality.

I can hear my readers say, "But the person is not convinced that the cause has been removed."

In the experience I refer to they were absolutely convinced, and in my next book there will be a fitting opportunity, I hope, to explain at considerable length this mental condition which seems so extraordinary and unreasonable.

This is one of the most difficult mental defects a teacher can be called upon to eradicate, because it shows that the person so afflicted is dominated by a subconsciousness built up of delusion and undue apprehension without any relation to common-sense or fact. Another instance of the disregard of reasoned judgment is demonstrated to me constantly in the mental attitude of my pupils when they first come to me for lessons. In the endeavour to perform some particular act, however simple, many pupils exhibit a degree of apprehension out of all proportion to the point at issue. This makes progress almost impossible and causes considerable distress. It is not my intention to deal with any of the complex examples which come to my notice in my daily experience with intelligent and educated pupils, but merely to set down some of the very simple examples of difficulties which seriously retard the progress of well-meaning people while undergoing any training.

Naturally a teacher is forced to point out at the beginning that this or that is wrong. All too frequently the pupil at once shows distinct signs of unnecessary apprehension. As this condition is the most retarding feature in any teaching work, I have for years in my own work devoted special attention to it and at once make an attempt to prevent it by endeavouring to put the pupil into "communication with his reason." There are numerous and widely differing means to this end in the early stages of reeducation to the description of which a whole book might easily be devoted, but it is sufficient here to mention it in a general way. I begin by pointing out that we expect these different things to be wrong, that their being so is not a case for worry or apprehension, seeing that they assuredly can be corrected. I draw attention to the obvious fact that a pupil comes to a teacher because there is something wrong. That must be the primary idea, otherwise the teacher's help is superfluous. Then, why worry when the defects or failings are discovered and made known to one? Surely it is something that should evoke pleasure rather than worry. In other words, if we have imperfections and defects, we seek help because we are conscious of their existence, because we wish to know definitely what they are, so that we may have an opportunity to eradicate them. Common-sense dictates that we should find a teacher who can detect these defects and diagnose their cause, and when this is done the pupil has much to ease his mind, much to bring him real satisfaction when the teacher can assure him of their eradication, and a changed mental attitude should immediately follow. But many people are so out of communication with their reason that it needs days of re-education to establish a satisfactory working basis.

Now, to bring about the correct performance of any act by the principles of my system of teaching it is not necessary at the beginning to call upon the pupil for any specific physical efforts. This very fact should remove immediately any cause for worry or apprehension, but in many cases it does not. When this is the case the teacher must explain that the reason that the pupil is unable to perform the act correctly is that he believes that there is something for him to do physically, when as a matter of fact the very opposite is necessary. He *is doing* what is wrong. Obviously he should begin then by ceasing to to do what is wrong, not by endeavouring blindly to do what is right. The process is this: Apprehensively he tries to do what he thinks his teacher desires him to do. The old wrong subconscious orders follow in their usual channels, and before he realizes the fact he is performing the act in the old wrong manner. Therefore he must learn to inhibit these incorrect subconscious orders, which result in undue physical tension and the imperfect use of his muscles. But instead of employing inhibition, he adds to his difficulties by renewing his efforts on the old basis to put right what he is told is wrong, and he actually employs increased force in accordance with his own estimate of the amount needed to perform the act. And why so? Chiefly because the ordinary human being has lost the habit of inhibition, and because he is guided here by his sense of feeling, in this connection the most unreliable guide.

When it is explained to such a pupil that inhibition is the first step in his re-education, that his apprehensive fear that he may be doing wrong and his intense desire to do right are the secrets of his failure, he will invariably endeavour to prevent himself from doing anything, by exerting force usually in the opposite direction. And so he creates a second harmful force which, in conjunction with the first, serves only to increase the undue physical tension and to intensify the already exaggerated apprehensive condition. The fundamental principle in the reeducation of such a subject is the prevention of this undue and unnecessary apprehension. He must not attempt to remedy any defect by "doing something" physically in accordance with his sensory appreciation, which is the outcome of his erroneous preconceived, ideas and incorrect psychophysical experience. His reasoning power is dominated by his sense of feeling where his psycho-physical self is concerned, so that he cannot even attempt to carry out any physical act except the one *he feels* to be right, despite the fact that by his reasoning faculties and practical proof he knows that his sense of feeling is misleading and is the outcome of erroneous preconceived ideas. We must therefore make him understand that so very frequently in re-education the correct way to perform an act *feels* the impossible way. There is only one way out. of the difficulty. He must recognize that guidance by his old sensory appreciation (feeling) is dangerously faulty, and he must be taught to regain his lost power of inhibition and to develop conscious guidance. The teacher must with his hands move the pupil's body for him in the particular act required, thereby giving him the correct kinesthetic experience of the performance of the act.

To the uninitiated this may seem a simple matter, but if my reader will put it to the test, it will not be necessary for me to convince him that it is quite otherwise in the majority of cases. This is not surprising when it is realized that as soon as the teacher places his hands on the pupil and attempts to move him, he is at once in contact with his faulty and deceptive sense of feeling, the dominating sense in the subconsciously controlled person in such circumstances. My experience has proved that the pupil at first will act in precisely the same way if I attempt to perform the act for him as if I had asked him to do it without my assistance. He is just as apprehensive as a result of one request as of the other, and in this state of apprehensiveness he is, mentally and physically, impossible to deal with from the standpoint of re-education. He conjures up in his mind all kinds of fears that he will do this or that incorrectly. If you mention that he did a certain thing when you placed your hands on him, he will make an endeavour physically to prevent himself the next time. This, of course, is one of the worst errors a pupil can make. It is usually attended by far more tension and apprehension than when he performed the act which you pointed out was incorrect. The re-education work really begins here, and it takes weeks, nay, sometimes months to bring the pupil to a stage in his co-ordination when he will be really once more in communication with his reason. With these facts before us I feel that my reader will advocate with me the necessity of adopting principles which will create new and correct habits, and eradicate needless apprehension and fear from the souls of human beings. To this end we must break the chains which have so long held them to that directive mental plane which belongs to the early stages of his evolution. The adoption of conscious guidance and control (man's supreme inheritance) must follow, and the outcome will be a race of men and women who will outstrip their ancestors in every known sphere, and enter new spheres as yet undreamt of by the great majority of the civilized peoples of our time. The world will then make in one century greater progress in evolution towards a real civilization than it has made in the past three.

CHAPTER VI - INDIVIDUAL ERRORS AND DELUSIONS

FREQUENT reference has already been made to individual delusions, errors, and misconceptions of a more or less harmful nature associated with our mental and physical efforts in the different rounds of daily life. I wish now to draw special attention to those which may be said to have a more strictly personal bearing than those referred to heretofore, and which have not been fully recognized despite the fact that they are forerunners of unusually harmful and persistent bad habits. The individual misconceptions, errors, and delusions to which I refer are indicated in the cases which follow. They are the direct result of most laudable attempts to accomplish something considered necessary to the welfare of life, something which seemed essential to success in life, something which was felt to be a worthy achievement in life. Among these I would instance:

The attempt to bring about some change considered necessary in the shape or use of a part or parts of the physical organism, and to conceal or change some supposed or real psycho-physical peculiarity, weakness, or defect.

The clinging to erroneous reasoning, in the face of undoubted evidence which revealed the errors in such reasoning, regarding the mode of procedure adopted in the attempt to prevent or "cure" attacks of illness and painful or disagreeable experiences. The decision that a certain condition is present, and the definite conclusion as to its degree of harmfulness or the extent of its general effect upon the organism, or its influence upon the daily conduct of life.

The attempt to remedy what the subject considers a lack of concentration.

The attempt to gain benefit by relaxation in consequence of the recognition of undue tension of the muscular mechanisms, not only in physical acts, but also during the attempt to rest by sitting in a chair, lying on a bed or couch, etc.

The detection by the subject of symptoms which are always considered serious and call for immediate eradication and future prevention. The original conception in this connection is influenced by warped and incorrect subconscious experiences, and consequently a narrow and perverted view is taken of the conditions present.

The "one-brain-track" method is in operation, and the *modus operandi* adopted by the subject is therefore deduced from false premises. Symptoms are considered causes, and furthermore the chief aim of the subject in practical procedure is the attainment of the "end" desired, not the due and proper considered analysis of the "means whereby" which will secure that "end."

Perusal of the following history of cases will serve to draw attention to the little-recognized but all-important fact that mankind's attempts at self-help on a subconscious basis in the spheres indicated cause him to live in a self-created danger zone. Moreover, the area of this zone is being gradually but surely extended by each and every new experience in those psychophysical activities where attempts are being made in what may be termed preventive and curative spheres.

The foregoing applies to a very wide range of bad habits over the whole organism, such as:

(1) The cultivation of harmful habits in consequence of misdirected energy and mental delusions which cause disorders and defects of the eyes, ears, nose, and throat, etc.

(2) The development of the dangerous habit of not hearing any instructions, opinions, advice, or argument which if put into practical procedures would be contrary to the psycho-physical subconscious habit associated with some defect, peculiarity, or other abnormal condition.

(3) The development of over-compensation in some direction. "Running an idea to death," as we say.

(4) The harmful domination by a "fixed idea," on account of which the subject struggles to gain an "end" without adequate and sound consideration of the correct "means whereby," or of possible consequences to him in the cultivation of defects during this process.

CASE I
An attempt to hide a thin neck.

The subject's wife intimated that the thinness of his neck made him look many years older than his real age. This occupied his mind for some time and he was increasingly worried by his wife's statement. He felt that he must find a practical remedy, but in the plan which he

conceived he thought only of the "end" he had in view, which was to
hide what he believed to be an unsightly and unsatisfactory part of his
anatomy. He conceived the idea of wearing as high a collar as
possible and, not being satisfied with the results, he took a second
and very harmful step in the hiding plan. This was a deliberately
cultivated habit of shortening his neck until the under part of the
jaw rested on the top of the collar, while the head was pulled back until
the lower part of the back of the head pressed on the back of the collar.
From his point of view a satisfactory remedy had been found and the
denounced neck was at last concealed from view.

In the standing, sitting, and walking positions these uses, or
rather misuses, of the muscles of the neck soon grew into a very
firmly established habit which became associated with a general
tendency towards the shortening of the neck and spine, whilst the
muscular co-ordinations of the whole organism were gradually and
harmfully interfered with.

Some of my impressions at the first interview were:
(1) The exaggerated rolling movement of his body when walking.
(2) The pressure of the under part of the jaw and the lower part
    of the back of the head or upper part of the neck on the
    collar.
(3) The marked lumbar curve of the spine with the usual shortening
    of stature and protruding abdominal wall. Harmful flaccidity
    of the abdominal muscles and general stagnation of the
    abdominal viscera.
(4) The fallen arches of the feet—one foot caused very
    considerable pain at times when standing or walking.
(5) That colour of the skin and condition of the eyes which
    indicates serious internal disorder.
(6) The upper part of the front of the chest was held unusually
    high (pouter-pigeon style). The thorax was harmfully rigid.
(7) The apprensive mental condition in his own personal affairs and
    also in his contact with the practical affairs of life.

His medical advisers were unanimous in declaring that he was
suffering from nerve and digestive disorders, and he failed to make
any improvement during many years of treatment. In his own words,
he "had year by year gone from bad to worse," until he was often too

nervous to cross a street with ordinary traffic, and his fears in this connection were increased by frequent attacks of giddiness, when he almost lost his sense of equilibrium. He complained of painful distention after meals and suffered much from insomnia.

CASE II
An attempt to conceal his height when interviewing actor-managers of shorter stature.

It is well known in professional circles that there is a prevailing idea in the mind of the actor-manager that he should be taller than the actors who support him. The actor to whom I refer in this instance discovered that he had missed several lucrative engagements by being taller than the actor-manager with whom he had arranged personal interviews. Incidentally I may mention that he possessed a fine physique and enjoyed at this time good health. It is obvious that an actor must endeavour to prevent the loss of good engagements in his profession, and as his height was the only stumbling-block to his desires and necessities, he considered his problem from this point of view only. Never for a moment did it occur to him that any mental or physical harm could result. With this *"one idea"* view he sought his remedy, and soon decided that he must train himself to use his mechanism in such a way that he could shorten his stature during interviews when seeking professional engagements. He succeeded in this direction, but unfortunately subconscious guidance and control take no head of the "means whereby" to be employed. His idea was merely to make an effort to gain the "end" he desired, and he was never really conscious of the actual means he ultimately employed. He merely conceived the idea of standing in a way which made him appear as short or even shorter than the person he was interviewing. Of the real mechanical happenings he was quite ignorant, and he had never thought it necessary to improve his knowledge in these all-important processes. This man came to me for help some four or five years after beginning to adopt this way of standing during the interviews. He had then been suffering for a considerable time from loss of voice, general exhaustion, and nerve and digestive disorders. On one occasion he experienced a mental and physical crisis which his medical advisers called "a nervous breakdown."

Some of my impressions at the first and subsequent interviews were:

(1) The undue and harmful lumbar curve of the spine with the corresponding intra-abdominal pressure.

(2) The harmful and undue depression of the larynx and its accessories.

(3) The exaggerated "gasping" in breathing in vocal and dramatic efforts.

(4) The undue rigidity of the thorax and a minimum intra-thoracic capacity.

(5) The lack of mental control in any attempts in psycho-physical re-education and co-ordination.

(6) A pessimistic mental outlook with recurring fits of depression.

(7) In the standing and walking positions the hips were held too far forward, the knee joints were pressed too far back, and the angle of the torso from the hips was harmfully inclined backwards, with a general tendency, as we say, to narrow the back.

CASE III
A fixed idea regarding a definite mode of procedure adopted after experiencing a week's illness in bed.

This lady developed certain symptoms for the first time. She then decided upon a practical common-sense method of dealing with them which would undoubtedly have been the correct one in the long run. The day following her first efforts in this direction her feeling-tones registered that she was much worse, in fact that she was very ill indeed, and that the latest symptoms were worse than those she had hoped to remove and ultimately prevent. She decided that her attempted remedy had actually been the cause of additional trouble, without in the least relieving the original symptoms. The remedy referred to was one of activity, mental and physical. She therefore came to the conclusion that this new phase of her illness had been actually brought about by the attempt she had made to fight her symptoms by simple but active methods. This conclusion became with her an *idee fixe*.

In discussing the matter the foregoing facts were vouchsafed to me. She said that she had given due consideration to them and had concluded in consequence of her experiences that the real remedy must be to go to bed and to allow the disorder to take its own course. This unfortunate experience caused her to continue to hold the idea that as soon as she felt any of the symptoms which preceded the first attack she should at once go to bed, to "prevent," as she put it, "the possibility of increasing the severity of the attack." She was absolutely convinced that she must not make any effort, mental or physical, in the way of removing or resisting the disorder as she had done on the first occasion of the attack. She decided upon the easy way of inactivity and non-resistance. Once the conscience seized upon an excuse for what the mental and physical "make-up" really craved she was doomed, and her conclusions were really influenced by this subconscious tendency. It is not surprising that after pursuing such a mistaken course for six months the attacks became more frequent and severe despite medical help, and the periods during which she was confined to her bed, and which she considered necessary to her recovery, became longer and longer. But the worst feature in her case was her increasing inability to make a real effort in the direction of health. She was actually developing her tendency to allow things to take their course, she was cultivating the serious habit of being guided and controlled by what she "felt" rather than by her reason. Her relatives at last came to the conclusion that her psycho-physical condition was serious, and I was asked to express an opinion from this point of view.

At the outset one suspected some incorrect and harmful mental outlook, and after a few lessons succeeded in securing the pupil's admission of the fact. A review of this mental conception may prove interesting and perhaps of great value to my readers, as it shows that as long as it existed her chances of permanently eradicating these symptoms were nil. The whole procedure constituted a prostitution of those physical, mental, and spiritual forces which are inseparable from and absolutely essential to that condition of the human organism which we call good health. This lady was suffering from the inadequate functioning of the vital organs associated with and responsible for good digestion and adequate elimination. This was proved conclusively by the results which accrued from a method of psycho-physical treatment which restored the adequate functioning after the eradication of the mental conception referred to above.

The position then was as follows:

Certain symptoms were recognized which were the result of the stagnation of organs which needed increased activity in functioning. As a matter of fact they happened to be such as would have yielded more or less to a steady walk of a mile or so daily. The effect, therefore, of lying in bed for days was only a palliative measure. But in consequence of her first impressions through her debauched sense of feeling when she adopted active measures as a remedy, she made a definite decision against their adoption in the future; in fact, she absolutely objected to a second trial of the active method. In the intervals of freedom from these attacks the one idea was rigidly held in mind that on the recognition of the slightest symptom she must go to bed and remain there. She even considered any other mode of procedure harmful. These ideas became an obsession. She became less and less in communication with her reason, and the fact that she admitted that the attacks became more frequent and the symptoms more serious did not cause her to relinquish her bed treatment in favour of some other. The fact is that her debauched emotions and feeling-tones had taken control instead of remaining secondary factors to reason.

It is possible to give hundreds of such cases, and attention is specially drawn to the fact that the *one idea* principle of meeting life's difficulties is the real cause of these serious results. If Case I, for instance, had held in his mind the "means whereby" for the concealment of his neck and had watched carefully the effect of his attempts in this particular upon his whole organism, he would assuredly have come to the conclusion that the thin neck, natural in his case, was to be preferred to the positive evils he was unconsciously cultivating. Neither he nor his wife detected any of the numerous defects as they developed during the neck-concealing process. On the other hand, they were both aware that he was gradually failing in health and had reached a stage which his medical advisers considered serious. Of course, never for a moment was the influence of the process of shortening the neck connected with his increasing troubles and disorders. His mental training had been solely on the lines of working for an "end" ("one-brain-track method") instead of holding in his mind the "means whereby."

He had never doubted for a moment the fallibility of the sensory appreciation of his organism. He firmly believed that immediately he decided to effect a change in his physical self he could command it by the employment of his subconscious guiding principles. He was unaware that these instinctive factors were delusive and unreliable as his directive agents.

If the reader's interest can be aroused in this connection, all-important benefits must accrue in even the simplest spheres of daily life. Furthermore, the more difficult problems of living will be sensibly considered without fear of the disastrous results which are now so common.

CHAPTER VII - NOTES AND INSTANCES

SINCE this book was published in this country, I have received a steady flow of letters from interested readers, lay and professional, which have been of great value to me. Among this correspondence three pertinent questions occur again and again, and I am forced to infer (1) that these points are of peculiar interest to my readers and (2) that no satisfactory explanation of them is suggested by the application of the broad principles I have laid down. I feel, therefore, that in this edition it may be well to treat these questions and various other matters which arise out of them for the benefit of future readers.

The three main questions—two of which occur in about eighty per cent of the letters I have received —are these:

(1) What is the correct standing position, and the position of mechanical advantage?

(2) How is the reader to apply the principles of conscious control, as here laid down, to specific bad habits such as over-indulgence, whether in tobacco, alcohol, particular foods, etc., or to the cure of such diseases as asthma, tuberculosis, constipation, spinal curvature, appendicitis?

(3) What are the outward signs of improvement to be noted during treatment, and are there scientific reasons for these results? In this connection I have several times been asked to give particulars of some of my more striking and representative cases.

I will take these three questions *seriatim,* and devote as much space as possible to each of them.

"What is the correct standing position, and the position of mechanical advantage?"

I think the average man is very apt to forget that he cannot assume a position of stable equilibrium and a position which ensures a perfect mobility, unless his feet are so placed as to furnish at once a stable pose and a ready pivot and fulcrum.

The most perfect base is obtained by setting the feet at an angle of about forty-five degrees to one another. In all other erect positions (the defects becoming exaggerated as this angle is decreased) it will be found that there is a tendency to hollow and shorten the back and to protrude the stomach, and if any effort is made to avoid these serious faults in posture, such effort will only result—unless the feet are moved to the correct position—in a stiffened, uneasy, and unstable attitude. It is not possible, however, to set out in written language the correct pose of the feet and legs in the ideal standing position, and I therefore subjoin four photographs which have been specially taken for this purpose (first published on 22nd October, 1910), and which show quite clearly not only the correct position of the feet, the fundamental problem, but also how the whole body of the person is thereby thrown into gear.

But when this ideal position is realized, the task of obtaining it by each individual has still to be undertaken. With reference to this task, I cannot do better than quote my pamphlet of July, 1908, entitled *Why "Deep Breathing" and Physical-culture Exercises Do More Harm than Good*, from which it will be clearly seen that the ideal position varies slightly according to the idiosyncrasies of the person concerned. The passage in question is as follows:

In the first place, to allow a pupil to assume, of himself, a certain standing position, means that his own perceptions and sensations are given the sole onus of bringing about the co-ordination upon which such standing position depends, an onus which they are quite unable to bear.

The perceptions and sensations of all who need respiratory and physical re-education are absolutely unreliable. It is the teacher who should have the responsibility of certain detailed orders, the literal carrying out. of which will ensure for the pupil *what is then the correct standing position for him.* I emphasize this last, because no one stereotyped position can be correct for each and every pupil. When the person so employs the different parts of his body that one can speak of his 'harmful position in standing or walking,' it is only by causing the physical machinery gradually to resume correct and harmonious working, thus changing the position from time to time, that serious harm can be averted and satisfactory results secured. I may point out, moreover, that in trying to assume the 'proper standing position' at the outset, the pupil unavoidably puts severe strain upon the throat, thereby paving the way for throat, ear, and eye disorders."

Matthias Alexander

Take the case, for example, of a boy who stoops very much, and combines a sinking above and below the clavicles with abnormal protrusion of the shoulder-blades. If he is told to "stand up straight" he will at once make undue physical effort to carry out the order thus crudely given, with the result that the shoulders will be thrown backward and upward, the shoulder-blades still further protruded, and the front and upper parts of the chest unduly elevated and expanded. There will also be a narrowing, a sinking, and a flabbiness of the lower dorsal and posterior thoracic region, with corresponding fixed protrusion and rigidity of the front chest wall, undue arching of the lumbar spine, shortening of the body, and harmful stiffening of the arms and neck, instead of a fullness, broadness, and firmness of the back, with free mobility of the chest walls, resulting in normal curve of the lumbar region and comparative lengthening of the spine. With the arms hanging vertically, the relative position of that part of the thorax where the lungs are situated will be seen to be in front of the arms, instead of being, as it should be, behind them. In such a position, the boy feels helpless, and tires rapidly, owing to the imperfect co-ordination, and any attempt to accustom him to this erect posture will ultimately result in deterioration rather than improvement.

Now the narrowing and arching of the back already referred to are exactly opposite to what is required by nature, and to that which is obtained in re-education, co-ordination, and readjustment, viz., *widening of the back and a more normal and extended position of the spine.* Moreover, if these conditions of the back be first secured, the neck and arms will no longer be stiffened, and the other faults will be eradicated.

In order to obviate the evils enunciated in the last two postulates, the teacher must himself place the pupil in a position of mechanical advantage,[22] from which the pupil, by the mere mental rehearsal of orders which the teacher will dictate, can *ensure the posture specifically correct for himself,* although he is not, as yet, conscious of what that posture is.

------

[22] See also note, Part I, Habits and Thought of the Body.

I further elaborated the same point in *Why We Breathe Incorrectly* (November, 1909), and from this pamphlet I will now quote another passage which bears directly on some important points involved, viz.:

"There can be no such thing as a ' correct standing position ' for each and every person. The question is not one of correct position, but of correct co-ordination (i.e., of the muscular mechanisms concerned). Moreover, any one who has acquired the power of co-ordinating correctly, can readjust the parts of his body to meet the requirements of almost any position, while always commanding adequate and correct movements of the respiratory apparatus and perfect vocal control—a fact which I demonstrate daily to my pupils. Continual readjustment of the parts of the body without undue physical tension is most beneficial, as is proved by the high standard of health and long life of acrobats. It is a significant fact that the very reverse is the case with athletes, showing that undue muscular tension does not conduce to health and longevity."

From what I have now said, it will be quite evident that the primary principle involved in attaining a correct standing position is the placing of the feet in that position which will ensure their greatest effect as base, pivot, and fulcrum, and thereby throw the limbs and trunk into that pose in which they may be correctly influenced and *aided* by the force of gravity. The weight of the body, it should be noted (see diagram AA), rests chiefly upon the rear foot, and the hips should be allowed to go back as far as is possible without altering the balance effected by the position of the feet, and without deliberately throwing the body forward. This movement starts at the ankle, and affects particularly the joints of the ankles and the hips. When inclining the body forward, there must be no bending of the spine or neck; from the hips upwards the relative positions of all parts of the torso must remain unchanged. When the position is assumed, it is further necessary for each person to bring about the proper lengthening of the spine and the adequate widening of the back. The latter needs due psycho-physical training such as is referred to in the two extracts quoted above.

This standing position as now explained is physiologically correct as a primary factor in the act of walking. The weight is thrown largely upon the rear foot, and thus enables the other knee to be bent and the forward foot to be lifted; at the same time the ankle of the rear foot should be bent so that the whole body is inclined slightly forward, thus allowing the propelling force of gravitation to be brought into play.

The whole physiology of walking is, indeed, perfectly simple when once these fundamental principles are understood. It is really resolved into the primary movements of allowing the body to incline forward from the ankle on which the weight is supported and then preventing oneself from falling by allowing the weight to be taken in turn by the foot which has been advanced. This method, simple as it may appear, is not, however, the one usually adopted. The mechanical disadvantage displayed in what is known as a "rolling gait," for instance, a gait which is common enough, is absolutely impossible when the instructions given are carefully followed. And the effect upon the whole mechanical mechanism of the person concerned is shown by the fact that when the coordinating principles brought about by this method are established, there is a constant tendency for the torso to lengthen, whereas the usual tendency—due to faulty standing position and the incorrect co-ordinations which follow—is for the torso to shorten.

Nearly every one I examine or observe in the act of walking employs unnecessary physical tension in the process in such a way that there is a tendency to shorten the spine and legs, by pressing—if I may so put it familiarly—down through the floor instead of, as it were, lightening that pressure by lengthening the body and throwing the weight forward and moving lightly and freely. In consequence of the "shortening" and "pressing down" just referred to, the civilized peoples are becoming more and more flat-footed. The properly co-ordinated person employs a due amount of tension in such a way that the tendency of the spine and legs is to lengthen, and the equilibrium is such that the undue pressure through the floor is absent, and there is a lightness and freedom in the movements of such a person that is most noticeable. The person who is flat-footed has only to establish these conditions to restore the natural arch of the flat-foot.

We can find, perhaps, no better instance of the necessity for the application of the principles of conscious control to these fundamental and essential propositions of standing, walking, and running, than in the photographs taken of Dorando as he appeared when he was making his last terrible efforts to reach the tape at the conclusion of the Marathon race in London in 1908. One sees that he was desperately wearied, and that whatever conscious control of his muscular mechanisms he may ever have obtained, he was at this moment completely under the domination of subconscious (or subjective) control, that he was out of "communication with his reason." His body, as we see him in these photographs, is thrown back from the hips, his arms are outstretched behind him, and his legs are bent forward at the knee. As a consequence, he is compelled to use almost all his physical force in order to save himself from falling backwards. He is struggling against a tremendous gravitational pull which is dragging him away from his goal. If Dorando, magnificent athlete as he undoubtedly was, had been trained in the principles of conscious control, such an attitude would have been impossible for him, tired and exhausted even as he was. For if he had not been subconsciously controlled, he would have employed his commonsense at this moment and would have acted according to the guidance of its mandate. It is at such critical moments that we have urgent need for the control of reason, for it is then that we suffer most from the loss of the animal equivalent— instinct.

Dorando's muscles may have been taxed to their utmost capacity, but if he had been consciously controlled he would have leaned forward, not back, and while he had the strength necessary (but a very small part of the strength he was actually expending) to prevent himself from falling on his face, that gravitational force would have dragged him on instead of dragging him back from the object of his achievement, as was actually the case. He would, in short, have been able to make the *best* instead of the *worst* use of his powers.

Faults such as we see exaggerated in this instance are to be found in the carriage of many people to-day, and the fact is one of great importance to medical men. Patients are constantly advised to take walking exercise, although in many cases that exercise undoubtedly does more harm than good. In my opinion it is very essential that all doctors should devote more attention to this subject than they are devoting at the present time, in order that they may be in a position to advise which of their patients will be benefited by taking walking exercise, and which of them by so doing will aggravate the troubles from which they are suffering. For it should be evident, I think, that the good effects of fresh air and gentle exercise will be practically nullified if the patient can only obtain them by exaggerating and perpetuating the defects which have led him to the prescription.

These same rules are equally applicable in principle to the acts of sitting and of rising from a sitting position. Very few people have the right mental conception of the "means whereby" of these acts or of the correct use of the parts which should be employed in their performance, and this despite the fact that we are performing these acts continually, and with such apparent ease from our own point of view. If you ask any of your friends to sit down, you will notice, if you observe their actions closely, that in nearly all cases there is undue increase of muscular tension in the body and lower limbs; in many cases the arms are actually employed. As a rule, however, the most striking action is the alteration in the position of the head, which is thrown back, whilst the neck is stiffened and shortened. Now I will describe the correct method, but it must be borne in mind that it is useless to give what I here call "orders" to the muscular mechanism, until the original habit and the principle of mental conception connected with this action have been eradicated. If, for instance, before giving any of the "orders" which follow, the experimenter has already fixed in his mind that he is to go through the performance of sitting down, *as that performance is known to him,* this suggestion will at once call into play all the old vicious co-ordinations, and the new orders will never influence the mechanisms to which they are directed, because those mechanisms will already be imperfectly employed, and will be held in their old routine by the force of the familiar suggestion. Firstly, then, rid the mind of the idea of sitting down, and consider the exercise and each order independently of the final consequence they entail. In other words, study the "means," not the "end."

Secondly, stand in the position already described as the correct standing position, with the back of the legs almost touching the seat of the chair.

Thirdly, order the neck to relax, and at the same time order the head *forward* and up. (Note that to "order" the muscles of the neck to relax does not mean "allow the head to fall forward on the chest."

The order suggested is merely a mental preventive to the erroneous preconceived idea.)

Fourthly, keep clearly in the mind the general idea of the lengthening of the body which is a direct consequence of the third series of orders.

And fifthly, order simultaneously the hips to move backwards and the knees to bend, the knees and hip-joints acting as hinges.

During this act a mental order must be given to widen the back.

When this order is fulfilled, the experimenter will find himself sitting in the chair. But he is not yet upright, for the body will be inclined forward, unless he frustrates the whole performance at this point by giving his old orders to come to an upright position.

Sixthly, then—and this is of great importance— pause for an instant in the position in which you will fall into the chair if the earlier instructions have been correctly followed, and then, after ordering the neck to relax and the head forward and up, the spine to lengthen, and the back to widen, come back into the chair and to an upright position by using the hips as a hinge, and without shortening the back, stiffening the neck, or throwing up the head.

The act of rising is merely a reversal of the foregoing. Draw the feet back so that one is slightly under the seat of the chair, allow the body to move forward from the hips, always keeping in mind the freedom of the neck and the idea of lengthening the spine. Let the whole body come forward until the centre of gravity falls over the feet, that is to say, until the poise is such that if the chair were removed at this point, you would be left balanced in the position of a person performing the "frog dance," then, by the exercise of the muscles of the legs and back, straighten the legs at the hips, knees, and ankles, until the erect position is perfectly attained.

If you care to experiment on a friend in this act of rising, you will observe that in the movement as performed by an imperfectly co-ordinated person the same bad movements occur, tending to stiffen the neck, to arch the spine unduly, to shorten the body, and to protrude the abdominal wall. This completes the co-ordinating idea with regard to standing, walking, and sitting, and the exercises indicated in the explanations I have made will be found exceedingly helpful as a first step towards a proper and healthful use of the muscular mechanisms in these simple acts of everyday life.

Matthias Alexander

II.   *"How are the principles of Conscious Control to be applied to
the cure of specific bad habits, or to the cure of specific diseases?"*
The following letter is typical of many:

"Dear Sir,—I have read your book, *Man's Supreme
Inheritance,* with much interest, and I hope you will forgive me
if I venture to point out a difficulty which presents itself to my
mind, and probably to the mind of the ordinary reader.

"It is this: In what way is it proposed to *apply* the principle
of 'conscious control' in a given case—say in the overcoming of
a habit, such as smoking, to take a common example—or in the
case of functional disorders, as constipation? It seems to me that
the great attraction to most people of the popular books on so-
called 'New Thought' is that they lay down clear and precise rules
which can be put into practice, so that the reader knows what
he must do to be saved. But I confess I am unable to gather how
you would recommend setting about the attainment of your
principles. It would be a great help to me, and no doubt to others,
if this could be explained, and probably in the larger work which
you contemplate this will be more fully done.

In the meantime, however, if it is not asking too much, I should
be extremely grateful to you if you could very kindly indicate the
method you propose by which the principles could be applied in
such cases as I have suggested...."

Now, I may be doing the writer of this letter an injustice, but
I am inclined to class him among the many inquirers who seem
confidently to anticipate a miracle. In my introduction I have said,
"In this brochure will be found no mention of royal roads, panaceas,
or grand specifics," yet I feel sure that some of my readers have,
nevertheless, imagined that by some marvellous means they may be
cured by taking thought, despite all that I have written with regard to
that procedure. We see in one paragraph of the letter quoted above
a nice example of the desire to lean towards any mechanical method.
"The great attraction... of the popular books on so-called 'New
Thought,'" we read, "is that they lay down clear and precise rules
which can be put into practice." It is true that I have not laid down
any "clear and precise rules" which may cover every conceivable form
of physical and mental trouble, as do the exponents of "New

Thought" and "faith-healing," and I think that my reason should be plain enough, for in my experience I have never found two cases exactly alike, and the detailed instructions which I might lay down for A might be extremely detrimental to B or C.

Nevertheless, since I see that some further explanation is needed, I will adumbrate the general principles which embrace the rule of application, however diverse the method may be in practice.

In the first place, all specific bad habits, such as overindulgence in food, drink, tobacco, etc., evidence a lack of "control" in a certain direction, and the greater number of specific disorders, such as asthma, tuberculosis, cancer, nervous complaints, etc., indicate interference with the normal conditions of the body, lack of control, and imperfect working of the human mechanisms, with displacement of the different parts of that mechanism, loss of vitality and its inevitable concomitant, lower activity of functioning in all the vital organs. When the subject has arrived at this condition, harmful habits become established, and the standard of resistance to disease is seriously lowered.

To regain normal health and power in such cases, what I have called "re-education" is absolutely imperative. This treatment begins, in practically all cases, by instructions in the primary factors connected with the eradication of erroneous preconceived ideas connected with bad habits, and the simplest' correct mental and physical co-ordination. The displaced parts of the body must be restored to their proper positions by re-education in a correct and controlled use of the muscular mechanisms. In this process the blood is purified, the circulation is gradually improved, and all the injurious accumulations are removed by the internal massage which is part and parcel of the increased vital activity from such re-education.

Thus the first stage in the eradication of bad habits and disorders is reached when improved conditions of health are established. Nor must it be forgotten that in this process of reeducation a great object lesson is given to the controlling mind. In the very breaking up of maleficent co-ordinations or vicious circles which have become established, a new impulse is given to certain intellectual functions which have been thrown out of play. The reflex action which is setting up morbid conditions can only be controlled and altered by a deliberate realization of the guiding process which is to be substituted, and these new impulses to the conscious mind have, analogically, very much the same effect as is produced on the body by the internal massage referred to above. The old accumulations of subconscious thought are dispersed, and room is made for new conceptions and realizations.

When the first stage is passed, it is just as easy at almost any time of life to establish "good" habits ("good," that is, by the test of all our experience and knowledge) as "bad" ones. Bad habits mean, in ninety-nine per cent of cases, that the person concerned has, often through ignorance, pandered to and wilfully indulged certain sensations, probably with little or no thought as to what evil results may accrue from his concessions to the dominance of small pleasures. This careless relaxation of reason, in the first instance, makes it doubly difficult to assert command when the indulgence has become a habit. Sensation has usurped the throne so feebly defended by reason, and sense, once it has obtained power, is the most pitiless of autocrats. If we are to maintain the succession that is our supreme inheritance, we must first break the power of the usurper, and then re-establish our sovereign, no longer dull and indifferent to the welfare of his kingdom, but active, vigilant, and open-eyed to the evils which result from his old policy of *laissez-faire*.

So many people, I find, seem to regard the principles of conscious control as a kind of magic which may be worked by some suitable incantation. They appear to think that we may obtain conscious control of, say, the secretive glands, that we may be able to give an order to secrete more or less bile or gastric juice by a command of the objective mind. If such a thing were possible, and if I could endow any person with such power to-morrow, I should know perfectly well that I should, by so doing, be signing that person's death warrant; I might equally well give him a dose of poison. To refer to my metaphor of the sovereign ruler, you might as well expect a king to order and superintend the detail of his subjects' private life as expect the conscious mind directly to order and. superintend every function of the body. If the king will ordain good and just laws, his policy will prosper; the detail of organization must be left to inferior officers. In the care of the body the organization is there, aptly and perfectly adjusted to its functions, and when the ruling power of conscious control has ordained the sane laws which shall establish peace and prosperity within the assembly, the organization already in force will work in harmony to its fit and proper ends. On the other hand, there is great danger in underrating the power of conscious control, which, if it must not be prematurely forced and made to intrude on automatic functions, must in no way be undervalued or delimited.

For instance, though it may not be possible to control directly each separate part of the abdominal viscera, we can control directly the muscles of the abdominal wall which encloses the viscera, and in reducing a protruding abdomen we can control many other muscles, notably those of the back, which when they are properly employed and co-ordinated will, by widening and altering the shape of the back, make place for the protruded stomach, allow it to occupy the natural position from which it has been ousted, and so give free play once more to the natural functions of the viscera that have been distorted and pinched by the forced positions they have had to assume. Here we see that though conscious control does not affect by a process of direct command, as it were, the lower automatic functions, there is great danger in assuming that such functions are beyond the reach of my methods.

This danger was brought before me when I read, in the *British Medical Journal* for December, 1909, an article on one side of my teaching contributed by Dr. S, an old pupil of mine. In this article Dr. S says:

> "Man's education does not always demand conscious instruction; in the absence of unfavourable circumstances he can learn by unconscious imitation of good models."

Now this is not demonstrably untrue, but at the same time it is, as I shall show, extraordinarily misleading, and is, in effect, just as valuable as the prescription of champagne and hothouse grapes for a pauper patient.

In the first place, we must remember, and has himself admitted the fact, that the normal is the rarest of all states. Medical experts find that their most constant source of error in diagnosis arises from the over-readiness to assume normal conditions in patients whose internal economies and muscular co-ordination are, in fact, far from the ideal standard of proportion and interdependence. Yet if the expert trained in physiology fails to note the distortions which are upsetting the whole economy, what body is to be named the supreme authority that shall select the "good models" for unconscious imitation?

In the second place, we have to reckon with a psychological factor which at once determines the question of the validity of unconscious imitation. This factor is the demonstrable truth that unconscious imitation does in nine hundred and ninety-nine cases out of a thousand lay hold of the faults of the imitated and pass over the virtues. In a long experience of re-educating many professional men and women for the stage in this country, I have had abundant opportunity to observe the methods of the "understudy" set to "imitate" his or her principal, and my invariable experience has been that subconscious imitation has always been shown by a reproduction of the actor's or actress's most prominent failings. The intellectual reading of the part, the subtler inflections of voice and the finer details of gesture are passed by, and the "understudy" reproduces the "mannerisms," all those obvious tricks of speech, manner, and gesture which are the least essential factors in the true reading of the part. Again, my experience in cases of stammering has shown me very clearly that, especially among boys and young men, the stutter has in a very large majority of cases come about by the imitation of some other boy. We do not find boys so apt to imitate one of their fellows who speaks particularly well.

Now this imitation of a fault in speech is subconscious and will not always right itself naturally, and the reason for this will become clear with a little consideration. Set a man to work on an elaborate and intricate piece of machinery. Tell him that if he moves a switch here and a lever there certain effects will be produced and certain desired results obtained. The movements are simple ones, and the man left to himself will be able to control the working of the machine with ease and certainty. But let us suppose that some essential part of the machine is put out of gear, and that the machine, instead of running smoothly and easily, begins to jerk and hiccough. Our assumed operator is immediately at a loss. He sees that there is something wrong, and that there is obvious friction where there was ease before; noise has taken the place of silence; but he knows nothing of the working of the machine save the elementary movements of the switch and lever, in the uses of which he has had instruction. Now, he may perform these movements again and again; but the machine still stutters, and our operator, quite at a loss, can do nothing to obviate these faults. He must allow the machine to continue working badly, if it works at all.

The boy we have adduced as an example of a stammerer, who has copied some fault of another boy and found that fault become permanent, is in exactly the same position as the unskilled operator of our illustration.

This boy knows the ordinary uses of his vocal machine, which have heretofore produced normal results, but he does not know enough of the machine to repair it when it is put out of gear; he cannot control the machinery so that it may at once be restored to its previous efficiency.

But just as the unskilled operator may be instructed in the complete mechanism he is set to supervise, and may then stop the machine when any fault becomes evident, discover the source of the defect, and set it right; so will any person who has been instructed in the principles of conscious control be able to detect and obliterate any fault in his vocal or any other bodily mechanism, even if that fault was originated below the level of consciousness.

These marked examples furnish a sound and unfailing analogy to the principles of unconscious imitation in their application to physiology. The perfectly co-ordinated man or woman does, as a matter of fact, offer less mark for imitation to the ordinary observer than the man or woman who displays an obvious defect, just as the perfectly dressed man or woman passes with less remark than those people who affect some exaggeration of costume in order to attract attention. Were we able at this time to set the Greek model before our children, we should be able to display it only on occasion, and the unconscious imitative powers of the child would seize hold far more readily of the marked defects with which it would be forced into contact during the greater part of its waking life. In a perfect world, unconscious imitation would not be able to exert a perverting influence, and to the conception of such a world we may well turn our attention, but we shall never attain it by any means other than these principles of conscious, reasoning, deliberate construction, or reconstruction, upon which I have based the whole of my theory and practice.

And, finally, there is still a serious danger to be reckoned with, even should we find sufficient methods in our present civilization from which we might learn by unconscious imitation. We must remember that during the advance of civilization mankind has lost the faculty we call instinct, the faculty which guided mankind in a state of nature as it still guides the lower animal world. During our advance from this primitive condition, the one great defect in our mental, physical, and educational training has been the failure to recognize that civilized life is the death-bed of instinct, and that in civilized life man's education must always demand conscious instruction. For we see that it is at the critical moments that men fail to rise to the occasion. In such a case as that of Dorando, already cited, we see that a perfectly trained athlete, a man capable of the magnificent effort he made in the great Marathon race, was robbed of his victory by his dependence at the critical moment on unconscious control as opposed to the conscious control which is the thesis of *Man's Supreme Inheritance.* And every day we are told that at critical moments, at the crisis of a debate, when suddenly called upon to decide a question of moment, or when faced with terrifying physical danger, men "lose their heads"—and fail. It is more especially at these times, at the crises of life, that the men who had been *educated* in the principles of conscious control would be capable of acting with the same reason and common-sense that characterized their mental and physical acts on the ordinary occasions of life. If they had relied upon *unconscious* imitation they would still be dependent, to a certain degree, on instinct.

Before leaving Question II, however, I will deal specifically with two of the prevailing maladies of our time, viz., spinal curvature and appendicitis, and show how the principles I have enunciated have a particular bearing on the prevention and cure of these two serious ailments.

1. Spinal Curvature. A perfect spine is an all-important factor in preserving those conditions and uses of the human machine which work together for perfect health, yet there are comparatively few people who do not in some form or degree suffer, perhaps quite unconsciously, from spinal curvature.

The present attitude towards this very serious mark of physical degeneration would be ludicrous were it not that the matter is one of almost tragic importance, and I may quote in this connection a letter of mine which appeared in the *Pall Mall Gazette* for 14th

March, 1908. After dealing with certain other matters which need not be reproduced here, I cited the following instances of the results of our present attitude:

"In our schools and in the Army, human beings are actually being developed into deformities by breathing and physical exercises. I have before me a book on the breathing exercises which are used in the army, and any person reasonably versed in physiology and psychology, and knowing they are inseparable in practice, will at once understand why so much harm results from them. Take either the officers or the soldiers. In a greater or less degree the unduly protruded upper chests (development of emphysema), unduly hollowed backs (lordosis), stiff necks, rigid thorax, and other physical eccentricities have been cultivated. It is for these reasons that heart troubles, varicose veins, emphysema, and mouth breathing (in exercise) are so much in evidence in the Army. As this is a matter of national importance, I am prepared to give the time necessary to prove to the authorities (medical or official) connected with the army, the schools, or the sanatoria that the 'deep breathing' and physical exercises in vogue are doing far more harm than good, and are laying the foundations of much graver trouble in the future. The truth is that all exercises involving 'deep breathing' cause an exaggeration of the defective muscular coordination already present, so that even if one bad habit is eradicated, many others, often more harmful, are cultivated.

"In this connection it is only necessary to point to the serious effects of 'deep breathing' and physical-culture exercises in the causation of throat and ear disorders, following upon the undue and harmful depression of the larynx—the crowding down of the structures of the throat—such depression occurring with every inspiration, and as a rule with every expiration. This disorganization and consequent strain in the region of the throat is always found exaggerated, and tends gradually to increase in people who are subject to asthma, bronchitis, and hayfever, and the removal of the factors causing such strain and disorganization means great relief and gradual progress towards the eradication of these disorders; but of course, all organic troubles should be removed in such cases."

Now I may say further that I have not, up to now, examined any method of physical-culture or respiration which has not tended to bring about in time some form of directly harmful lumbar spinal curvature. And I have never examined a case of the (alleged) cure of spinal curvature in which the front of the chest has not been harmfully altered, and very often seriously deformed. The original idea in diagnosis of spinal curvature which has led to the methods producing these results is "that the activity of the muscles is necessary to the retention of the spine in an erect position, in consequence of which, therefore, the primary cause for the scoliosis must be sought in an abnormal function of the muscles influencing the spine." This is the myopathic theory of Eulenburg, an authority whose dicta have had an important influence in medical practice.

The error of advocating physical exercises, as generally understood, of any kind in the treatment of spinal curvature is even greater than in the case of John Doe, whom I cited in the earlier part of this work and whose case should be again referred to in this connection. The question here also is one of correct conscious recognition, and it is much more marked in the case of spinal curvature than in the case of my earlier illustration, a case in which there was no special deformity, and in which the muscle-tensing exercises I deprecated did not work to emphasize a marked structural malformation.

The important factors in relation to spinal curvature are these:

(a) The bent or curved and therefore shortened spine.
(b) The decreased internal capacity of the thoracic cavity.

Plainly, attention must first be given to straightening and lengthening the curved and shortened spine. This can be done by an expert manipulator who is able to diagnose the erroneous preconceived ideas of the person concerned, and cause the pupil to inhibit them while employing the position of mechanical advantage. And it can be done without asking the pupil to perform what he understands as a single physical act. Moreover, if the correct guiding orders are given to the pupil by the teacher, and the pupil makes no attempt to hold him or herself in the lengthened position, such use of the muscular mechanism will, nevertheless, be brought about as will ensure that the torso is held in a correct position. Formerly the consciousness in regard to the correct action has been erroneous, a mere delusion, and the muscular mechanisms have worked to pull the body down. The truth of the matter is that in the old morbid conditions which have brought about the curvature the muscles intended by Nature for the correct working of the parts concerned had been put out of action, and the whole purpose of the re-educatory method I advocate is to bring back these muscles into play, not by physical exercises, but by the employment of a position of mechanical advantage and the repetition of the correct inhibiting and guiding mental orders by the pupil, and the correct manipulation and direction by the teacher, until the two psycho-physical factors become an established psycho-physical habit.

During this process of re-education, factor *(b)* has not been forgotten. A little consideration will show that any alteration in the spine must necessarily affect the position and working of the ribs. (The analogy of the keel of a boat and the ribs which spring from it may well be held in mind to make clear the following explanation.) It will be seen that as the ribs are held apart by muscular tissues (analogous to the boards of a boat), a bending of the spine will not buckle the ribs unless great force is applied, force sufficient to rupture the muscular tissue. But it is equally evident that there must be some play in the ribs in order that they may adjust themselves to the new position. This play is effected in the human body (and would be effected mechanically in the ribs of a boat, if they possessed sufficient elasticity) by the coming together of the ends of the "false" and "flying" ribs—that is, those lower ribs which are not attached to the bony sternum. This flattening of the curve of the ribs and the approach of their free ends towards each other reduce the thoracic cavity, just as in our illustration of the boat its capacity would be reduced if we forcibly narrowed the distance between the thwarts. On the other hand, we see that by increasing the thoracic capacity, and so increasing the distance between the ends of these ribs, we are applying a mechanical principle which by a reverse action tends to straighten the spine.

These two actions—the re-education of the "Kinaesthetic Systems" and the increasing of the thoracic capacity which applies a mechanical power by means of the muscles and ribs to the straightening of the spine—are both aspects of the one central idea, and are not separate and divisible acts.

2. *Appendicitis.* The prevalence of appendicitis has always seemed to me one of the most striking proofs of the inefficiency of present-day methods in regard to health. At times I am filled with wonder that we permit such bad conditions to become established as may necessitate the removal of the appendix. It is, of course, well known that the operation is frequently performed when the conditions do not warrant such extreme measures, but cases have come under my notice, nevertheless, and those not among the uneducated classes, in which the symptoms had become so aggravated by years of harmful habits of life as to necessitate the major operation. Fortunately there is a section of the medical profession which objects, on scientific grounds, to the removal of the appendix in all but extreme cases, and this opposition and the evidence adducible as to the comparative ease with which the exaggerated condition may be avoided and the trouble completely cured by natural means, are doing much to limit the sphere of those champions of the knife who are never content unless they can be dissecting the living body.

There can be no question or shadow of doubt that when the whole frame is properly co-ordinated and the adjustment of the body is correct and controlled according to the principles I have enunciated, it is a practical impossibility to get appendicitis. The cause of the trouble is due to imperfect adjustment of the body which allows or forces the abdominal viscera to become displaced and to fall. The first consequence of this is a change of pressures and the loss of the natural internal massage, present in normal conditions. This leads to constipation, among other symptoms, and permits the gradual accumulation of toxic poisons.

When the trouble has already shown itself and there is some positive inflammation of the appendix and tenderness in that region, it is by no means too late to apply my methods. The new co-ordinations which may in such cases be brought about very quickly, and established later, at once relieve false internal pressures and permit a natural readjustment of the viscera, and the furtherance of a rapid return to a healthy and normal condition is greatly accelerated by the internal massage.

With regard to this latter treatment, to which I have already referred in this chapter, I may mention that many pupils have asked me if I use internal massage in my system of re-education. In my brochure on the *Theory and Practice of Respiratory Re-education,* included in Part III of this book, it will be found that I used this description, as I said, for lack of one that was sufficiently comprehensive, but the principle itself is one of the first importance.

When a patient or pupil is placed in the position of mechanical advantage I have so often had occasion to refer to, the manipulator can secure the maximum movement of the abdominal viscera in strict accordance with the laws of nature, and will obtain at the same time a maximum functioning of all the internal organs. In this way foreign accumulations are dissipated, constipation is relieved, and the more or less collapsed viscera—the cause of all the trouble—are restored to their proper places and resume their natural functions.

All these things, it will be seen, are essential factors in the prevention and cure of appendicitis, and I may add that the application of these principles in a very large number of cases in which an operation has been medically advised has conclusively demonstrated their value to the individual and to the race.

Appendicitis,, like influenza, is probably almost an impossibility in the natural state; it is one of the results of civilization and subconsciously controlled mechanisms, and is possible only through the conditions we have developed; and these adventitious troubles and ailments will continue to appear and to do their work of destruction until some general recognition is made of the necessity for substituting conscious control for the partly superseded forces which in a wild state render these ailments impossible.

III. *"What are the outward signs of improvement to be noted during treatment?"*

The signs of improvement are manifold and they necessarily vary according to the nature of the original defect, but I will set out here some of the more characteristic, such as occur in generally typical cases.

We see, in the first place, that the characteristic defects of the body, whether displacements of some part or parts of the muscular mechanism (in some cases even displacement of the bones), or defects of pose which throw some unusual strain upon a muscle, or, more commonly, a group of muscles not intended to take such strain, all have some correlated defects, which may be observed by the instructed as certain visible peculiarities and abnormalities. And we must draw particular attention in this connection to the fact that these outer signs are *correlated* with the inner defects. Neither outer sign nor inner defect is from one point of view the *result* one of the other. The original cause is some faulty or imperfect co-ordination or conception of function; the inner defect and outer sign-mark are equally a consequence as they are to us an index.

As we should naturally expect, the chief sign-manual is to be found in the face. To me, that is a most valuable document upon which are written many curious, intricate, sometimes alarming confessions. The expression of the eyes, the set of the lips, the drawing of the forehead, and the more pronounced dragging of the flexible face muscles, are all marks which may be read by the expert, and, to answer the question directly, one of the earlier outward signs of improvement is to be found in a relaxation of the forced and unnatural expression which results from these contortions. It must be obvious that I cannot here set out in detail the symptomatic distortions which accompany the various internal defects, but one may be noted as an exemplar for the others, however diverse.

The case in question was one of dilation of the heart, and as such was brought to me by a medical friend, and, as a matter of fact, though this was the most alarming symptom, it was but one of many springing from deep-seated causes. Incidentally I may note that the spine was arched inwards, the legs were unduly and most abnormally stiffened when the patient was in a standing position, and the upper part of the chest was held most harmfully high—this last symptom being the influence which produced what was really a tertiary effect, though in this case the most threatening one—viz., the dilation of the heart. Now this patient carried certain very curious marks in the face: first a general expression of strain in the eyes and cheek muscles, and secondly four very marked indents or pits in the forehead. Here, indeed, were marks which the expert might read, and it was extremely interesting to note, as my treatment progressed and the patient recovered the proper use of the body and a consequent return to perfect health, first, the disappearance of the strained expression of eyes and face muscles, and secondly, the gradual filling up of the four curious indentations in the forehead. In this case the original symptoms were so marked that the patient's friends all commented on the change of expression during the progress of the treatment.

The face, however, is by no means the only index. Many defects lead, by way of stiffened neck and throat muscles, to an alteration in the quality and power of the voice. There, too, the mode of movement and the failure to express purpose in muscular action, the fumbling, indirect attempt to perform a simple act, are aids to diagnosis, either of the original defect or, by their reversion to natural, easy functioning, of the progress of the cure.

Generally, also, we observe a clearing of the skin and eyes as the defects are eradicated, improvements which are due to better circulation and the improved quality of the blood, factors which bring about a continually increasing power in the organism to purge itself not only through the bowels and kidneys, but also through the skin.

Lastly, we may note a general improvement in physique, in the carriage of the body, in the whole appearance of coordinated, reasoned control.

Another curious and interesting test of the co-ordinated person who is attaining conscious control of the uses of his body is obtained by observing his hands when they fall to his sides in the position which comes naturally to him. One may say that there are three main stages to be observed in man's development in this particular, though the gradations are many and not, perhaps, always strictly progressive. The first stage may be observed in the lowest savages, the Hottentot, the Australian aboriginal, and many races at an early stage of development. Such examples stand with body thrown back from the hips, stomach protruded, and—here is the test—*with the palms of the hands forward,* the elbows bent into the sides, the thumbs sticking out away from the body. The second stage is evidenced in the average civilized man of to-day, who stands as a rule with the palms of his hands towards his body, his elbows to the back, his thumbs forward. In the third stage, the properly co-ordinated person stands with the back of his hands forward, the thumbs inwards, and the elbows slightly bent outwards. This is a curious but little-known test, which, in my experience, has never failed as an index to imperfect muscular co-ordination.

I believe I have now answered in sufficient detail the somewhat wide intention of these three main questions, but in conclusion I will note one further point that has been raised.

This is the question as to why the great majority of men and women breathe from their stomachs or the upper chest, and so allow, among other evils, the costal arch to be narrowed and the flying ribs to become constricted and stiffened. In the case of many women there can be no doubt that this is due to the use of tight corsets, which confine these ribs and do great general harm in constricting the natural play of the vital functions. But another and, in my opinion, the primary cause is the common practice of swathing a child in bands almost immediately after birth, and keeping him so fettered during many months of infancy. The idea of this practice is to prevent rupture in male children should they be subject to violent fits of crying or coughing, but the question of the relative tightness or looseness of these swathings is left in the hands of a nurse, who, in the great majority of cases, thinks it well to be on the safe "side" by winding the child unnecessarily tightly. Obviously the early habit is retained through life unless it is broken by some outside influence. The pliancy of the young organisms is such that the functioning of the breathing apparatus is quickly readjusted, but the evils which gradually accumulate, from this and similar causes, do not show themselves as a rule till much later in life.

Another cause is any imperfect adjustment of the muscular mechanism, a failure which may be due to incorrect training, to unconscious imitation, or to any of the chances which are always being presented to the child in the haphazard system of physical education which obtains in our nurseries and schools.

And on this note I may well conclude my chapter, for no argument I can advance in favour of a careful consideration of the principles I have laid down can have such cogency and force as the most superficial examination of the physique of the children in our schools and the adults in our streets. We are indeed suffering, not only in Great Britain, but on the continents of Europe and America, from a failure to recognize that man is no longer a natural animal, whose life-habits were dependent on the development of the faculty of instinct, and that all systems of physical-culture (and how diverse they are!) must necessarily fail unless they take into account that first and last essential, the free use and consciousness of the reasoning, controlling mind.

Matthias Alexander

PART III - THE THEORY AND NEW PRACTICE OF A OF RESPIRATORY METHOD RE-EDUCATION

First published 1907.

"Whoever hesitates to utter that which he thinks the highest truth, lest it should be too much in advance of the time, may reassure himself by looking at his acts from an impersonal point of view.... It is not for nothing that he has in him these sympathies with some principles and repugnance to others. He, with all his capacities, and aspirations, and beliefs, is not an accident, but a product of the time. He must remember that while he is a descendant of the past he is a parent of the future; and that his thoughts are as children born to him, which he may not carelessly let die."—HERBERT SPENCER.

INTRODUCTORY

IT may be of interest to my readers to know that the method I have founded is the result of a practical and unique experience, for my knowledge was gained—

1. While vainly attempting to eradicate personal, vocal, and respiratory defects by recognized systems.
2. While afterwards putting into practice certain original principles, which enabled me to eradicate these defects.
3. While giving personal demonstrations of the application of these principles from a respiratory, vocal, and healthgiving point of view.

I first imparted the method thus evolved to patients recommended by medical men over ten years prior to June, 1904. At that date I introduced it to leading London medical men, who, after investigation, decided that the method was, as one doctor put it, "the most efficient known to (him)."

The method makes for—

In Education

1. Prevention of certain defects hereinafter referred to.
2. Adequate and correct use of the muscular mechanisms

concerned with respiration.

In *Re-education:*

1. Eradication of certain defects hereinafter referred to.
2. Co-ordination in the use of the muscular mechanisms concerned with respiration.

The result of (2) is not only to make that function efficient, but also to ensure that normal activity and natural massage of the *internal organs* so necessary to the adequate performance of the vital functions and the preservation of a proper condition of health.

F. MATTHIAS ALEXANDER.

Matthias Alexander

THE THEORY OF RESPIRATORY RE-EDUCATION

THE artificial conditions of modern civilized life, among which is comparative lack of free exercise in the open air, are conducive to the *in*adequate use of breathing power. Indulgence in harmful habits of feeding and posture have caused these same habits, through heredity and unconscious imitation, to become "second nature" in the great majority of adults to-day and frequently in children, even at an early age.

The normal condition of vigour in the action of the component parts of the respiratory mechanisms is greatly interfered with; general nervous relaxation is brought about, and a feeble, flabby action becomes permanent.

Certain muscles of the thoracic mechanisms which should take the lead in the performance of the breathing movements remain entirely inert for the greater part of life, whilst others, which were never intended by nature to monopolize this particular act but only to serve as a relief or change, are used solely for the act of breathing.

Hence arises a condition in which the posture, the symmetry of the body, the graceful normal curves of the whole frame, suffer alteration and change.

The capacity and mobility of the thorax (chest) are decreased, its shape (particularly in the lumbar region, clavicles, and lower sides of the chest) is changed in a harmful way, and the abdominal viscera are displaced, whilst the heart, lungs, and other vital organs are allowed to drop below their normal position. Inadequate holding-space of the thorax—which means a distinct lessening of the "vital capacity"—and displacement of the vital organs within it, are great factors in retarding the natural activity of the parts concerned, which are therefore unable fully and naturally to perform their functions. In these circumstances the natural chemical changes in the human organism cannot be adequate.

The serious interference with the circulatory processes and the inadequate oxygenation of the blood prevent the system from being properly nourished and cleansed of impurities, for the action of the excretory processes will be impeded and the whole organism slowly but surely charged with foreign matter, which, sooner or later, will cause acute symptoms of disease.

It will at once be understood that the defects enumerated produce distinct deterioration in the condition of the different organs of the body, and it is well known that an organ's power of resistance to disease depends on the adequacy of its functioning power, which in its turn depends on adequate activity.

Records exist which prove that Chinese physicians as early as 2000 B.C. employed breathing exercises in the treatment of certain diseases. It is therefore obvious that the people concerned had reached:

1. A stage in their evolution which corresponds with that of our time, i.e., demanding re-education.
2. A stage of observation of cause and effect similar to that of to-day, which led them to see the need of reeducation. Such re-education is essential to the restoration of the natural conditions present at the birth in every normal babe, though gradually deteriorated under conditions of modern life.

In recent years the following members of the medical profession have urged the inestimable value of the cultivation and development of the respiratory mechanism, and their conclusions have been borne out by the practical results secured by respiratory re-education combined with proper medical treatment.

MEDICAL OPINIONS CONCERNING THE EVIL EFFECT OF INTERFERENCE WITH AND INADEQUATE USE OF THE RESPIRATORY PROCESSES

Mr. W. Arbuthnot Lane, surgeon to Guy's Hospital, in his lecture published in the *Lancet,* December 17, 1904, p. 1697, urges that reduction in the respiratory capacity is a very great factor in lowering the activity of all the vital processes of the body, and that in the first instance inadequate aeration and oxygenation is the result of a serious alteration in the abdominal mechanisms, and afterwards this insufficient aeration impairs the digestive processes. Dr. Hugh A. McCallum, in his clinical lecture on "Visceroptosis" (dropping of the viscera), as published in the *British Medical Journal,* February 18, 1905, p. 345, points out that over ninety per cent of the females suffering from neurasthenia (exhaustion of nerve force) are victims of visceroptosis, and that the conditions present are bad standing posture, imperfect use of the lower zone of the thorax, and the lack of tone in the abdominal muscular system which leads to defective intraabdominal pressure. He also mentions that Dr. John Madison Taylor of Philadelphia and Keith of England were the two first to point out that the origin of this disease begins in a faulty position and use of the thorax.

In a leading article in the *Lancet,* December 24, 1904, 1796, this passage occurs:

"Whatever may be the causes, it is certain that an increasing number of town-dwellers suffer from constipation and atony of the colon, and that purgatives, enemata, and massage are powerless to prevent their progress from constipation to coprostasis."

CONVALESCENTS

The value of respiratory re-education in the treatment of convalescents was pointed out recently (1905) by M. Siredey and M. Rosenthal in a paper read at a meeting of the Societe Medicale des Hopitaux.

An excerpt from the *Lancet,* February 18, 1905, p. 463, reads as follows:

"They said that respiratory insufficiency was one of the causes of the general debility which showed itself after an acute illness. It was easily recognized by the following symptoms, which the patient presented, namely, thoracic insufficiency, shown by absence or impairment of the movement of the thorax; and diaphragmatic insufficiency, shown by immobility or recession of the abdomen during inspiration—a condition met with in pseudo-pleurisy of the bases of the lungs.

Respiratory re-education was, in their opinion, the specific treatment for respiratory insufficiency. In the case of convalescents it constantly produced a progressive threefold effect, namely, expansion of the thorax, diuresis, and increase of weight. It promoted in a marked degree the recuperation of the vital functions which followed acute illness, and the general health of the patients improved rapidly. It ought to be combined with other forms of treatment, and the action of the latter was enhanced by it."

The matter of preventing defective and restoring proper action clearly calls for attention. The foregoing will enable the reader definitely to understand what is necessary, viz.,

1. In *Prevention.* The inculcation of a proper mental attitude towards the act of breathing in children, to be followed by those detailed instructions necessary to the correct practice of such respiratory exercises as will maintain adequate and proper use of the breathing organs.

2. In *Restoration.* A body possessing one or other or all of the defects previously named will need re-education in order to eradicate the defects brought about by bad habits, etc., and to restore a proper condition. As the breathing mechanism is ordinarily unconsciously controlled, it is necessary, in order to regain full efficiency in the use of it, to proceed by way of conscious control until the normal conditions return. Afterwards, when perfected, unconscious control—as it originally existed prior to respiratory and physical deterioration—will supervene.

CHAPTER II - ERRORS TO BE AVOIDED AND FACTS TO BE REMEMBERED IN THE THEORY AND PRACTICE OF RESPIRATORY RE-EDUCATION

"Each faculty acquires fitness for its function by performing its function; and if its function is performed for it by a substituted agency, none of the required adjustment of nature takes place; but the nature becomes deformed to fit the artificial arrangements instead of the natural arrangements."—HERBERT SPENCER.

ANYTHING that makes for good may be rendered harmful in its effect by injudicious application or improper use, and many authorities have referred to this fact in connection with breathing exercises. For the guidance of my readers I will detail some of the harmful results which accrue from the attempt to take what are known as "deep breaths" during the practice of breathing and physical exercises, in accordance with the instructions set down and the principle advocated in recognized breathing systems.

At the outset let me point out that respiratory education or respiratory re-education will not prove successful unless the mind of the pupil is thoroughly imbued with the true principles which apply to atmospheric pressure, the equilibrium of the body, the centre of gravity, and to positions of mechanical advantage where the alternate expansions and contractions of the thorax are concerned. In other words, *it is essential to have a proper mental attitude towards respiratory education or re-education, and the specific acts which constitute the exercises embodied* in it, together with a proper knowledge and practical employment of the *true primary movement* in each and every act.

I may remark that I recognized this factor and put it to practical use over twenty years ago, but it has been quite overlooked or neglected in the other systems formulated before and since that time. In fact, when I introduced my method to leading London medical men they quickly admitted the value of this important factor, and expressed their surprise that on account of its importance it had not been previously advocated, seeing that from a practical point of view it is so essential, not only in the eradication of respiratory faults or defects (re-education), but also in preventing them (education).

A proper mental attitude, let me repeat, then, is all-important. From its neglect arise many of the serious defects ordinarily met with in the respiratory mechanism of civilized people, all of which are exaggerated in the practice of customary "breathing exercises"

1. *"Sniffing"* or *"Gasping."* If the "deep breath" be taken through the nasal passages there will be a loud "sniffing" sound and collapse of the alas nasi, and if through the mouth, a "gasping" sound. The pupil has not been told that if the thorax is expanded correctly the lungs will at once be filled with air by atmospheric pressure, exactly as a pair of bellows is filled when the handles are pulled apart.

It is a well-known fact, but one greatly to be regretted, that many teachers of breathing and physical exercises actually tell the pupils that, in order to get the increased air-supply they *must* "sniff."

Worse than this, many medical men are guilty of similar instruction to their patients, and when giving a personal demonstration of how a "deep breath" should be taken, they "sniff" loudly and bring about a collapse of the alae nasi, throw back the head, and interfere with the centre of gravity. Of course, it is only necessary to remind them of the law of atmospheric pressure as it applies to breathing, and they at once recognize their error.

Such a state of affairs serves to show that lamentable ignorance prevails even in the twentieth century in connection with so essential a function as breathing, and on reflection we must realize the seriousness of a situation which, from some points of view, is really pathetic.

Most people, if asked to take a "deep breath," will proceed to—I use the words spoken by thousands of people I have experimented upon—"suck air into the lungs to expand the chest," whereas of course the proper expansion of the chest, as a primary movement, causes the alae nasi to be dilated and the lungs to be instantly filled with air by atmospheric pressure, without any harmful lowering of the pressure.

2. During this harmful "sniffing" act it will be seen that—

(a) The larynx is unduly depressed; likewise the diaphragm.

The undue strain, caused by this unnatural crowding down of the larynx and its accessories, is undoubtedly the greatest factor in the causation of throat troubles, especially where professional voice-users are concerned. This has been abundantly proved by the practical tests which I have made during the past twelve years. My success in London with eminent members of the dramatic and vocal profession, sent to me by their medical advisers, might be mentioned in this connection.

(b) The upper chest is unduly raised, and in most cases the shoulders also.

(c) The back is unduly hollowed in the lumbar region.

(d) The abdomen is generally protruded, and there is an abnormally deranged intra-abdominal pressure.

(e) The head is thrown too far back, and the neck unduly tensed and shortened at a time when it should be perfectly free from strain.

(f) Parts of the chest are unduly expanded, while others that should share in the expansion are contracted, particularly the back in the lumbar region.

(g) During the expiration there is an undue falling of the upper chest, which harmfully increases the intra-thoracic pressure, and so dams back the blood in the thin-walled veins and auricles and hampers the heart's action.

(h) Undue larynx depression prevents the proper placing and natural movements of the tongue, the adequate and correct opening of the mouth for the formation of the resonance cavity necessary to the vocalization of a true "Ah."

It is well known that the tongue is attached to the larynx, and therefore any undue depression of the latter must of necessity interfere with the free and correct movements of the former.

(i) The head is thrown back to open the mouth.

This is a common fault, even with professional singers, but a moment's consideration of the movements of the jaw —from an anatomical point of view—will show that it? should move downwards without effort, and that it is not necessary to move the head backwards in order to effect the opening of the mouth by the lowering of the jaw, since, as a matter of fact, the latter movement will be more readily and perfectly performed if the head remains erect without any deviatory posture.

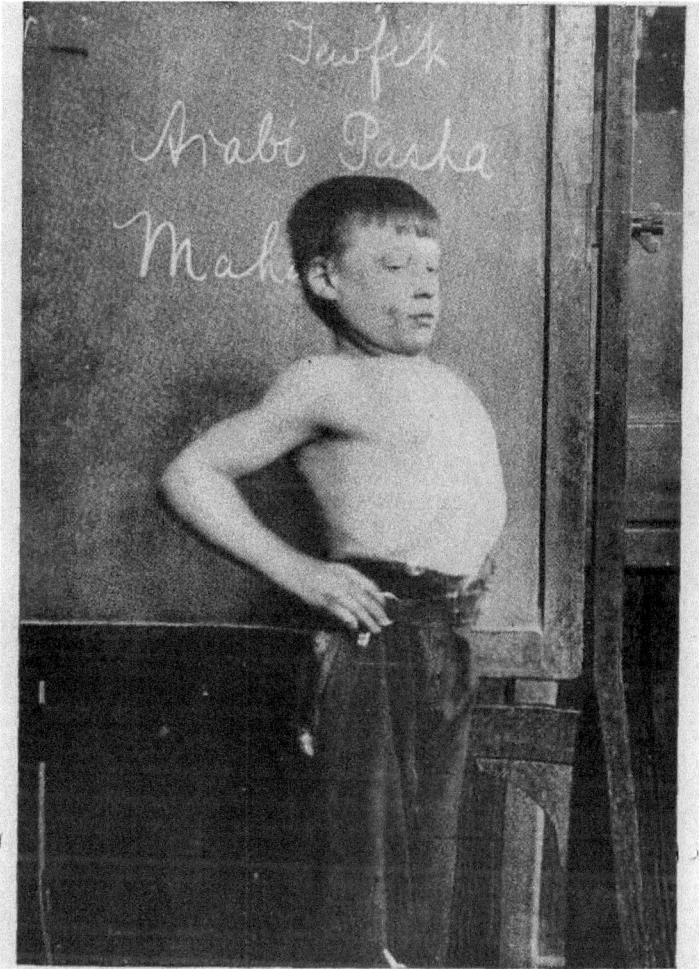

This photograph, published a few years ago in a daily paper, represents a member of a class in a London County Council School performing deep-breathing exercises. On the back of this page this lad may be seen at work in the class. These unfortunate boys as here shown are simply being developed into deformities. Luckily of late a change for the better has taken place in school calisthenics.

Matthias Alexander

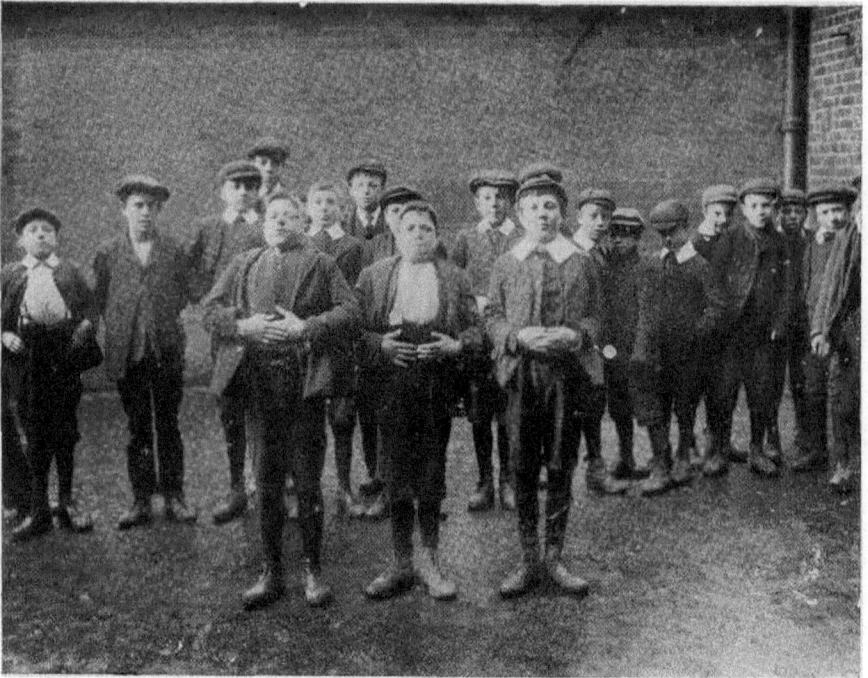

See note on previous illustration.

Every voice-user should learn to open the mouth without throwing back the head. Very distinct benefits will accrue to those who succeed in establishing this habit.

It is well known that the practice of "physical-culture" exercises has caused emphysema, and it has been suggested that unnatural breathing exercises have also been responsible for the condition. I refer to this because I wish to show that it would not be possible to cause emphysema by the method of respiratory education and re-education I have formulated.

Emphysema may be caused by:

1. The reduction of the elasticity of the lung cells and tissue resulting from undue expansion of the lungs and from their being held too long in this expanded position.

2. The undue intra-thoracic pressure, during an attempt at expiration or some physical act, upon the air cells, which remain filled with air in consequence of the means of egress from the lungs being temporarily closed by the approximation

of vocal reeds and ventricular bands.

If the fundamental principles of my method are observed, these conditions cannot be present during the practice of the exercises, and emphysema therefore not only cannot be produced, but is likely to be even remedied where previously existing.

In the first place, the tendency unduly to expand any part or parts of the thorax in particular, to the exclusion of other parts, is prevented by the detailed personal instruction given in connection with each exercise in its application to individual defects or peculiarities of the pupil. Moreover, the mechanical advantages in the body-pose and chest-poise assumed in these exercises cause them to be performed with the minimum of effort, and lead to an even and controlled expansion of the whole thorax. There is not, as is too often the case, an undue expansion of one part of the chest, while other parts, which should share in such expansion, are being contracted—a condition that obtains, for instance, when the diaphragm is unduly depressed in inspiration. In this latter case there is a sinking above and below the clavicles, a hollowing in the lumbar region of the back, undue protrusion of the abdomen, displacement of the abdominal viscera, reduction in height, undue depression of the larynx, and the centre of gravity is thrown too far back.

The *striking feature* in those who have *practised customary breathing exercises* is an *undue lateral expansion* of the lower ribs, when several or all of the above defects are present. This excessive expansion gives an undue width to the lower part of the chest, and there are thousands of young girls who present quite a matronly appearance in consequence. The breathing exercises imparted by teachers of singing are particularly effective in bringing about this undesirable and harmful condition.

The guiding principle that should be invariably kept in mind by both teacher and pupil is to secure, with the minimum of effort, perfect use of the component parts of the mechanisms concerned in respiration and vocalization. Then, sooner or later, adequate' mobility, power, speed, absolute control, and artistic manipulation must follow.

Most people—teachers as well as pupils—when thinking of or practising breathing exercises, have one fixed idea—viz., that of

Matthias Alexander

Causing a *great expansion* of the chest—whereas its proper and adequate *contraction* is equally important. There are, indeed, many cases in which the expiratory movement calls for more attention than the inspiratory.

Careful observation will show that those who take breath by the "sniffing" or "gasping" mode of breathing always experience great difficulty with breath-control in speech and song, or during the performance of breathing exercises. This remains true whether the air is expelled through the mouth or nasal passages, and it is due to the imperfect use of the thoracic mechanism, and the consequent loss of mechanical advantage already referred to at the end of the inspiration.

The natural and powerful air-controlling power is therefore absent, and its absence causes undue approximation of the vocal reeds, and probably of the ventricular bands in the endeavour to prevent the escape of air, which air, when once released

Under these conditions, is thereafter inadequately and imperfectly controlled.

In vocal use there is considerable increase in this lack of breath-control, the upper chest being more rapidly and forcibly depressed during the vocalization.

This is not a matter for surprise, for if a mechanical advantage is essential to the proper expansion of the thorax for the intake of air, it is equally essential to the controlling power during the expiration, and if during the expiration the upper chest is falling, it clearly proves that the advantage indicated is not present.

CHAPTER III - THE PRACTICE OF RESPIRATORY RE-EDUCATION

"If we contemplate the method of Nature, we see that everywhere vast results are brought about by accumulating minute actions."— HERBERT SPENCER.

HABIT IN RELATION TO PECULIARITIES AND DEFECTS

THE mental and physical peculiarities or defects of men and women are the result of heredity or acquired habit, and the most casual observer has noticed that certain peculiarities or defects are characteristic of the members of particular families, as, for instance, in connection with the standing and sitting postures, the style of walking, the position of the shoulders and shoulder-blades, the use of the arm, and the use of the vocal organs in speech, etc.

Such family peculiarities or defects are unconsciously acquired by the children, often becoming more pronounced in the second generation, such acquirements making for good or ill, as the case may be. I will, however, confine myself to an enumeration of those with a harmful tendency, as an understanding of bad habits is essential to the consideration of the teaching principles adopted in my method of respiratory physical re-education.

The chief peculiarities or defects may be broadly indicated as:

1. An incorrect mental attitude towards the respiratory act.
2. Lack of control over, and improper and inadequate use of, the component parts of the different mechanisms of the body, limbs, and nervous system.
3. Incorrect pose of the body and chest poise, and therefrom consequent defects in the standing and sitting postures, the interference with the normal position and shape of the spine, as well as the ribs, the costal arch, the vital organs, and the abdominal viscera.

Re-education, when one or other or all of these peculiarities or defects are present, means eradication of existing bad habits, and the following will indicate some of the chief ' principles upon which the teaching method of this re-education is based:—

That where the human machinery is concerned Nature does not work in parts, but treats everything as a whole.

That a proper mental attitude towards respiration is at once inculcated, so that each and every respiratory act in the practice of the exercises is the direct result of volition, the primary, secondary, and other movements necessary to the proper performance of such act having first been definitely indicated to the pupil.

It may prove of interest to mention that W. Marcet, M.D., F.R.S., and Harry Campbell, M.D., B.S., London, are of opinion that volition as such makes a direct demand upon the breathing powers, quite apart from all physical effort, and with these great advantages, that, unlike the latter, it neither increases the production of waste products nor tends to Cause thoracic rigidity, thus more or less retarding the movements of the chest.

The experiments made by Dr. Marcet show that the duration of a man's power to sustain the muscle contraction necessary to raise a weight a given number of times depends on the endurance of the brain-centres causing the act of volition rather than upon the muscular power.

An instance is quoted of a man who lifted a weight of 4 lb. 203 times, and who, after resting and performing forced breathing movements, raised the same weight the same height 700 times.

Regarding muscle development and chest expansion, Dr. Harry Campbell has in his book on breathing taken the case of Sandow. His conclusion will prove of interest. He pointed out that Sandow claimed to be able to increase the size of the chest 14 inches—that is, from 48 to 62 inches in circumference. Dr. Campbell then expressed the opinion that this increase is almost entirely the result of the swelling up of the large muscles surrounding the chest, and that most probably the increase in his bony chest (thorax) is not more than 2 to 3 inches, seeing that his "vital capacity" is only 275 cubic inches.

(For ten years past I have drawn the attention of medical men to the deception of ordinary chest measurements and to the evils wrought by the physical training and the "stand-at attention" attitude in vogue in the Army, and also to the harmful effects of the drill in our schools, where the unfortunate children are made to assume a posture which is exactly that of the soldier, whose striking characteristic is the undue and harmful hollow in the lumbar spine and the numerous defects that are inseparable from this unnatural posture.)

There is such immediate improvement in the pose of the body and poise of the chest whatever the conditions (excepting, of course, organized structural defects), that a valuable mechanical advantage is secured in the respiratory movements, and this is gradually improved by the practice, until the habit becomes established and the law of gravity appertaining to the human body is duly obeyed.

The mechanical advantage referred to is of particular value, for it means prevention of undue and harmful falling of the upper chest at the end of the expiration, which is always present in those who practise the customary breathing exercises, the pupil being then deprived of the mechanical advantage so essential to the proper performance of the next inspiratory act. Then follows due increase in the movements of expansion and contraction of the thorax until such movements are adequate and perfectly controlled.

Further, these expansions are primary movements in securing that increase in the capacity of the chest necessary to afford the normal oscillations of atmospheric pressure, without unduly lowering that pressure—or, in other words, they give opportunity to fill the lungs with air, while the contractions overcome the air pressure and force the air out of the lungs, and at the same time constitute the controlling power of the speed and length of the expiration.

The excessive and harmful lowering of the air pressure in the respiratory tract, and the consequent collapse of the alae nasi, is prevented by so regulating the respiratory speed that the lungs are filled by atmospheric pressure.

The value of this will be readily understood when it is remembered that such lowering, which is always present in the "sniffing" mode of breathing, causes collapse of the alae nasi. It also tends to cause congestion of the mucous membrane of the respiratory tract on the sucker system, setting up catarrh and its attendant evils, such as throat disorders, loss of voice, bronchitis, asthma, and other pulmonary troubles.

Matthias Alexander

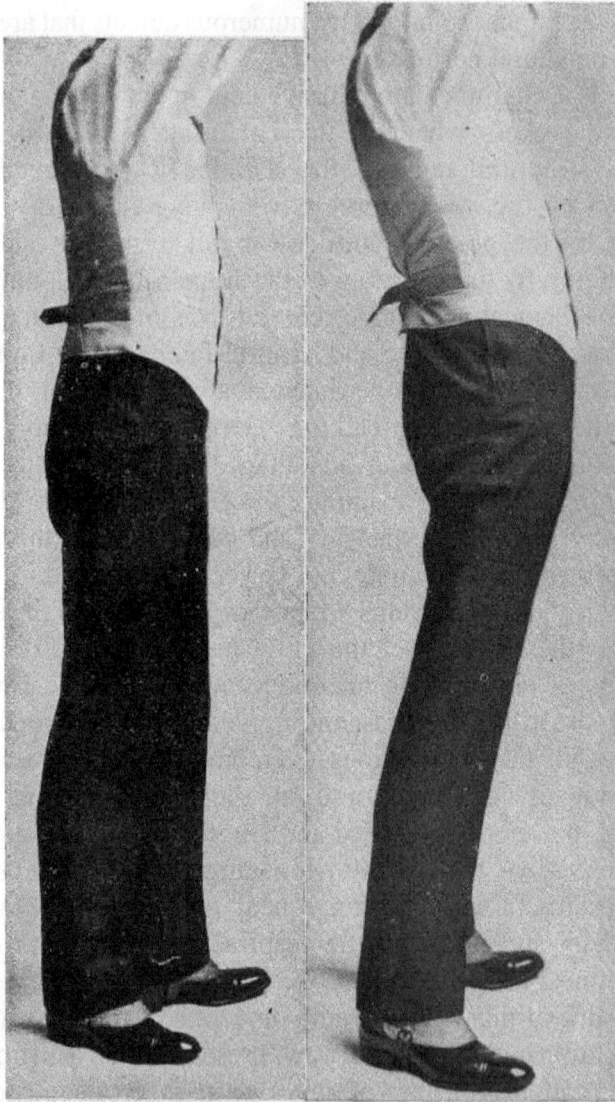

A *(Correct)*   **B** *(Incorrect)*

A—The feet are here placed in the ideal position for obtaining perfect equilibrium of the human machine, and for permitting the maximum activity of the functioning of the whole organism. NOTE.—It is evident that either the right or left foot may be in advance without affecting the correctness of the pose.

B—The feet are here placed in a position which compels an imperfect adjustment of the whole organism in order to secure even an imperfect equilibrium. This position results in the minimum activity of the vital functioning.

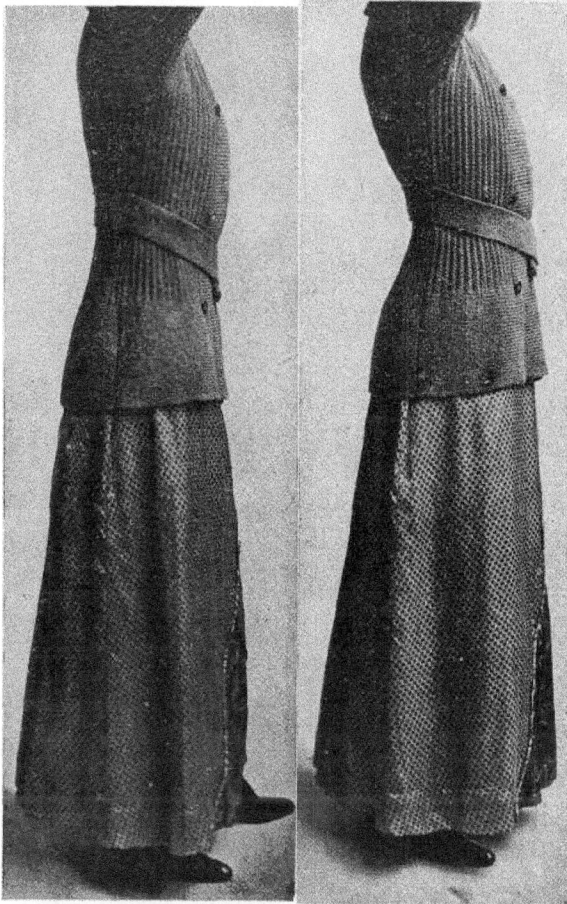

A *(Correct)*   **B** *(Incorrect)*

A—The feet are here placed in the ideal position for obtaining perfect equilibrium of the human machine, and for permitting the maximum activity of the functioning of the whole organism. NOTE.—It is evident that either the right or left foot may be in advance without affecting the correctness of the pose.

B—The feet are here placed in a position which compels an imperfect adjustment of the whole organism in order to secure even an imperfect equilibrium. This position results in the minimum activity of the vital functioning.

Matthias Alexander

From the first lesson the effect upon the splanchnic area is such that the blood is more or less drawn away from it to the lungs, and is then evenly distributed to other parts of the body. The intra-abdominal pressure is more or less raised, and there is a gradual tendency to the permanent establishment of normal conditions.

The use of bandages or corsets is to be condemned as treatment in protruding abdomen instead of the adoption of practical means to remove the cause. Such support to the abdominal wall is artificial and harmful, since it tends to make the muscles more flaccid. The respiratory mechanism should be reeducated, for this would mean a re-education or strengthening of the supports Nature has supplied. In other words, the sinking above and below the clavicles and the undue hollowing of the lumbar spine—the great factors in the direct causation of the protrusion of the abdomen—are removed, and a normal condition of the abdominal muscles established. This means a very decided improvement in the figure and general health.

The improvement in the abdominal conditions (the improved position of the abdominal viscera and the development of the abdominal muscles) is proportionate to that of the respiratory movements—a fact that can be readily understood when I point out that the movements of the parts are interdependent. When the faulty distention of the splanchnic area is present, it will be found that the diaphragm is unduly low in breathing; and when there is excessive depression of the diaphragm in respiration there is interference with the centre of gravity by displacement forward, and the compensatory arching backward in the lumbar region.

After a time there is such improvement in the use of the component parts of the mechanism that an inspiration may, if desired, be secured by a depression of the diaphragm, while at the same moment the condition in the splanchnic area is actually improved.

Improvement in respiratory exchange is secured by gradual increase in the expansions and contractions of the thorax, which increases the aeration of lungs, the supply of oxygen, and the elimination of CO_2.

The quantity of residual air in the lungs is greatly increased, and if the expired air is always converted into a controlled whispered vowel during the practice of the breathing exercises, very great benefits accrue, notably those derived from the prolonged duration of air in the lungs, and the proper interthoracic pressure necessary to force the adequate supply of oxygen into the blood and eliminate the due quantity of CO_2.

The employment of these whispered tones means the proper use of the vocal organs in a form of vocalization little associated with ordinary bad habits, and that perfect co-ordination of the parts concerned which is inseparable from adequately controlled whisper vocalization.

There is a rapid clearing of the skin, the white face becoming a natural colour, and a reduction of fat in the obese by its being burnt off with the extra oxygen supply.

This reduction in the weight and size is often quite remarkable, as also the development of the flaccid muscles of the abdominal wall and the consequent improvement in the activity of the parts concerned.

CONCLUDING REMARKS

THE foregoing will serve to draw attention to the far-reaching and beneficial effects of what, for the lack of a more satisfactory and comprehensive name, I refer to as respiratory re-education. It is a method that makes for the maintenance and restoration of those physical conditions possessed by every normal child at birth, the presence of which ensures a proper standard of health, adequate resistance to disease, and a reserve power which, if a serious illness should occur, will serve to turn the tide at the critical moment towards recovery.   The insurance of such a condition for a generation would mean the regeneration of the human race as constituted to-day; and I have no hesitation in stating that the results secured during the past twenty years, and particularly during the past thirteen years in London in co-operation with leading medical men, justify me in asserting that the practical application of the principles of this new method in education and re-education will be invaluable in overcoming the disadvantages and bad habits of our artificial civilized life, and that they will prove the great factor in successfully checking the physical degeneration of mankind.

INDEX

201, 203, 207

Body On Mind, 127

Boxing, 140

Breathing, 15, 33, 52, 55, 68,
87, 88, 89, 123, 132, 160, 165,
179, 186, 190, 191, 193, 194,
195, 198, 199, 200, 202, 203,
207

Bronchitis, 110, 179, 203

Brute Force, 97, 100, 101

Cancer, xi, 28, 110, 173

Catarrh, 203

Cause And Effect, 26, 58,
68, 70, 79, 120, 191

Chemical Changes, 27, 190

Chest, 89, 158, 166, 170, 180,
184, 186, 190, 195, 196, 199,
200, 201, 202, 203

Child, ii, xii, 14, 18, 42, 65, 66,
67, 68, 69, 70, 71, 72, 73, 74,
75, 76, 77, 78, 79, 80, 81, 82,
84, 87, 90, 91, 92, 93, 95, 99,
127, 177, 186, 209

Children, 24, 61, 63, 65, 66, 67,
68, 69, 70, 71, 72, 73, 75, 76,
77, 78, 79, 80, 84, 86, 90, 91,
92, 93, 142, 177, 186, 188, 190,
193, 201, 202

Circulation, xiii, 11, 173, 185

Civilization, 1, viii, xiii, 3, 4, 5,
6, 8, 16, 27, 41, 43, 50, 59, 66,
69, 71, 73, 75, 85, 86, 93, 95,
96, 97, 102, 105, 107, 109, 112,
115, 119, 137, 142, 143, 145,
155, 178, 183

Claim, 15, 22, 33, 77, 90, 101,
109, 110, 111

Colitis, 141

Colon, 11, 192

Common-Sense, 113, 151, 152,
153, 160, 178

Concentration, 53, 61, 62, 96,
103, 156

Confidence, ix, 38, 83, 100, 103,
108, 124, 129, 133

Conscious Guidance, viii, 5,
32, 34, 35, 40, 41, 43, 80, 83,
85, 86, 109, 112, 113, 115, 119,
120, 123, 125, 132, 135, 137,
141, 144, 145, 149, 151, 154,
155

Conscious Guiding, 127

Conscious Movement, 34

Consciousness, viii, 9, 15, 19,
23, 24, 25, 31, 39, 55, 56, 57,
85, 88, 118, 122, 128, 131, 138,
142, 149, 177, 181, 187

Constipation, 11, 141, 164, 172,
182, 183, 192

Contortions, 56, 137, 138, 139,
184

Control, 1, ii, iii, iv, v, vi, viii, xiv,
xv, 2, 5, 6, 7, 9, 10, 13, 14, 17,
18, 20, 21, 22, 24, 25, 26, 29,
30, 32, 33, 34, 35, 38, 39, 40,
41, 43, 44, 49, 50, 52, 54, 55,
60, 61, 63, 65, 68, 69, 70, 75,
77, 78, 80, 81, 83, 85, 86, 90,
92, 93, 97, 98, 102, 104,105,
107, 109, 113, 115, 119, 120,
122, 123, 125, 126, 127, 129,
131, 132, 133, 134, 135, 136,
137, 140, 141, 144, 145, 149,
150, 151, 155, 159, 160, 162,
164, 168, 172, 173, 174, 175,
176, 177, 178, 183, 185, 193,
199, 200, 201

Control And Co-Ordination, 55

Matthias Alexander

154, 173, 180
Predisposition, 30, 51, 59, 65
Prejudice, iv, 47, 59, 81
Pressing Down, 168
Proper Standing Position, 165
Psychology, 17, 18, 22, 87, 98,
    149, 179
Psycho-Physical, 35, 39, 41, 53,
    54, 69, 80, 86, 92, 97, 109, 115,
    117, 126, 127, 136, 145, 154,
    156, 157, 160, 161, 167, 181
Ralph Waldo Trine, 26
Reaction, iv, xv, 5, 17, 59, 73,
    104, 117, 138
Re-Adjustment, 35
Reason, xiii, 3, 14, 17, 18, 19, 20,
    28, 37, 40, 41, 42, 44, 46, 49,
    50, 51, 54, 57, 68, 71, 81, 85,
    87, 90, 96, 98, 99, 102, 103,
    110, 119, 123, 136, 145, 146,
    147, 149, 151, 153, 155, 161,
    162, 169, 173, 174, 176, 178
Re-Education, 13, 38, 42, 57, 83,
    89, 113, 120, 135, 153, 154,
    155, 160, 165, 166, 173, 181,
    183, 189, 191, 192, 193, 194,
    195, 198, 201, 207, 209
Reflex, 32, 53, 173
Reform, xv, 35, 36, 38, 47
Relaxation, ii, x, xi, 7, 13, 15, 53,
    57, 140, 156, 174, 184, 190
Resistance, xii, 59, 107, 111, 141,
    161, 173, 191, 209
Respiration, xiii, 68, 89, 180, 189,
    199, 202, 207
Respiratory, 11, 54, 65, 67, 121,
    126, 165, 167, 188, 190, 191,
    192, 193, 194, 195, 198, 201,
    202, 203, 207, 209

Responsibility, 72, 113, 165
Ribs, 181, 186, 199, 201
Rigidity, 26, 29, 30, 45, 46, 49,
    57, 121, 127, 128, 160, 166,
    202
Rome, 3
Rupture, 181, 186
Sandow, 202
School Furniture, 92
Science, x, xii, 17, 22, 29, 30, 63,
    65, 66, 125
Secondary Education, 84
Self-Hypnotism, 14, 31, 78, 98,
    130
Self-Preservation, 24, 59
Semi-Automatic, 9, 32
Sensation, 13, 27, 39, 41, 42, 68,
    114, 139, 174
Sensory Appreciation, 5, 14, 53,
    54, 124, 154, 163
Shortening, 77, 128, 134, 158,
    162, 166, 168, 171
Shoulders, 10, 13, 78, 79, 111,
    128, 166, 196, 201
Singing, 123, 140, 199
Sir Walter Scott, 61
Sitting, 15, 56, 57, 72, 156, 158,
    170, 171, 201
Skin, 22, 158, 185, 208
Speech, 31, 66, 68, 77, 80, 132,
    176, 200, 201
Spheres, 6, 34, 35, 37, 38, 40, 92,
    95, 97, 98, 99, 101, 104, 109,
    115, 155, 157, 163
Spinal Curvature., 178, 180
Spine, 114, 121, 122, 126, 128,
    134, 135, 158, 160, 166, 167,
    168, 171, 178, 180, 181, 182,
    184, 201, 203, 207

Matthias Alexander